The Step Up Diet

From Scratch...

The Quality, Quantity and Timing Solution to Childhood Obesity.

by

Marta Pin Muñiz Katalenas M.D.

To my children, all of them.

Table of Contents

Preface

When I first moved to the United States of America almost thirty years ago, my knowledge of the English language was very limited. I carried my English-Spanish dictionary with me at all times.

About one week after my arrival, I met the American man who would eventually become my husband, and we began dating. Our early conversations were full of misunderstandings and comical moments created by our language gap. A few months into our relationship (when I thought I was proficient in English), I decided to make him a chocolate cake for his birthday, something I was sure he was going to like. He tried a few bites, and looking at me with delight, asked how I had made the cake. I listed all the ingredients that my English permitted. Surprised, he exclaimed, "Ah, you made it from scratch!" This introduction to the phrase "from scratch" required a visit to my dictionary and some further explanation on his part.

One evening during the first months of our marriage, I was in bed miserable with the flu when my husband offered to make me some chicken soup. After a mere ten minutes, he returned to the room with a steaming concoction. When I was mystified at how he was able to prepare it in such a short time, he replied, "Oh, you thought I was going to make chicken soup from scratch?" He continued, "I just opened a can of Campbell's." This time, I was familiar with the expression, but the concept was still foreign to me. I had never thought about canned food as a possibility! I think I even felt a little offended; to me, opening a can was not a very considerate way to show affection for a sick person.

When it came time to choose a title for this book, it was clear what it had to be. These two words—*from scratch*—carry a lot of personal significance, and they also capture what I want to convey.

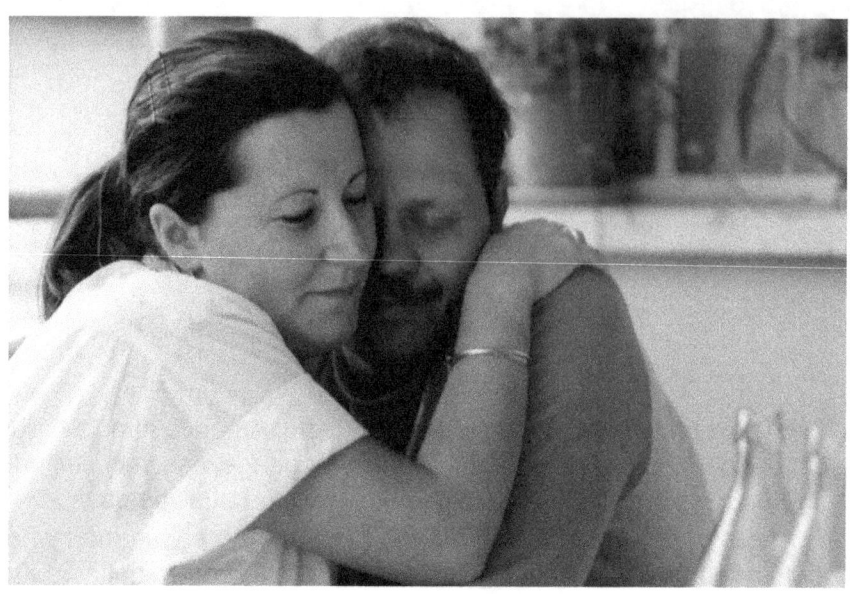

In order to begin, we must turn back the clock to examine the origins of the current obesity phenomenon in America. It is only for the last twenty-five to thirty years that our society has begun to gain consciousness about the issue. We began to realize that although we were eating "low fat" foods, our waistlines continued to expand as if not heeding the food labels. Then came the statistics reinforcing what we already knew: the typical American's body mass index (BMI) was on the rise, and with it, the prevalence of cardiovascular disorders and diabetes.

Now, a decade into the twenty-first century, we find ourselves witnessing the emergence of chronic disorders, previously diagnosed only in adults, in the pediatric population. We continue to scratch our heads, questioning, "How, with the most advanced medical technology on the planet and as the world's leader in medical research, could we possibly be responsible for this health-care disaster?"

Over the decades, the obesity phenomenon sneaked up on us gradually; it tipped our scales without setting off our radar. Coming out of the Great Depression, American families gathered around the table to share meals and thoughts. At the time, there was usually a household figure in charge of the grocery shopping and cooking. This figure was most often the mother, who had likely learned from her mother the art of preparing nutritious meals while providing variety and exposure to different food groups on a fixed budget. Eventually, that mother became the grandmother who continued fulfilling the role of the household shopper and cook. Those were the days when grandparents shared the house with their children and their children's families, or they lived near enough to help with the meal preparation.

As more females joined the workforce and families' lifestyles became more complicated, the family table suffered in quality. Shopping for nutritious ingredients gave way to convenience. When preparing dinner required too much time, it was easy to drive to the nearest fast-food joint where food was not only fast, but also cheap and available at any time.

We are now witnessing the emergence of the third generation of Americans addicted to fast-food and fad diets. In today's society where both parents work outside the home, there is no time to put any thought into the contents of the shopping cart. We shop for convenience without minding the amount of unhealthy additives we introduce into our bodies. We fill our pantries with processed foods, ready to ingest them without considering an alternative. In many cases, we don't even know there is an alternative.

When I decided to put my thoughts on paper and began to consider a title, I wanted it to summarize my message: we must fundamentally reconsider the quality of our health and eating habits, and we must learn how to choose the ingredients of our meals and to prepare them *from scratch*.

As a practicing pediatrician, I have been explaining my theories to my patients and their parents for the last twenty years. Thankfully, most of them understand, agree, and are able to improve the quality of their food choices in order to improve the quality of their lives. I hope you can, too. This plan is geared toward children and families who are learning good eating habits in order to avoid adulthood obesity.

So let's start *from scratch* ...

Acknowledgments

I would like to thank Melissa Shea, with IronDaisy.com, for the cover design and for her help with this book from the very beginning. I am also grateful to Bob Fullilove for copyediting and to Professor Toyin Falola for pointing me in the right direction.

And a special thanks goes to my niece, Elena Rodriguez Pin PhD, for her 24/7 technical support.

Introduction

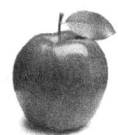 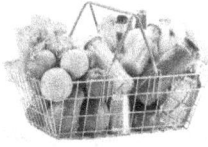 

Handling Obesity through

Quality,

Quantity,

and

Timing

Case Scenario: CJ

Let me tell you the story of a boy named CJ. He's like most any other healthy kid. He likes to play video games, but he also likes to get outside to play football or whatever his buddies are playing. He's not overly athletic or active, but he's not a total couch potato either.

Before school started, his mom took CJ to the pediatrician for his yearly wellness visit. His mom didn't expect anything to be amiss. CJ certainly didn't. He was a growing boy. He liked to eat and was husky for his age, but no one in CJ's family thought to be alarmed.

The pediatrician, however, noticed a marked increase in CJ's weight. It was becoming alarmingly disproportionate to the increase in his height. CJ all of a sudden was at risk of becoming obese.

When asked about changes in his eating habits, his mother related some changes in the family's routine. She explained that she didn't believe that leaving the house in the mornings on an empty stomach is a healthy idea, so she encourages CJ to eat a small breakfast at home. Because he qualifies for free school meals, he was eating a second breakfast when he arrived at school. Again, his mom thought that was a good idea because everyone knows you learn better when your stomach is full. Sometime close to noon, CJ would eat the school lunch. At 3:00 p.m., CJ was bussed to a local after-school program where, pretty much every day, he had a snack of granola bars (yes plural) and juice. When he got home at 5:00 p.m., his mother said that he was always hungry, but because she didn't want him to ruin his appetite for dinner, she gave him popcorn or fruit snacks with more juice in order to "tide him over" until dinner was ready.

CJ's mom thought that everything up to that point was as it should be. The only thing that did concern her was that when he finally got to the dinner table, CJ pushed aside the main course to make room for more side dishes. But because he didn't eat the main course, usually a meat dish, he was hungry again by 9:00 p.m., and so he finished off the day with some cereal in milk before bedtime.

CJ's parents didn't want to restrict the meals of a healthy, growing boy. They honestly believed his appetite was a result of increased demands related to his age. While his parents didn't like CJ eating only potatoes or rice for dinner with maybe some corn or peas, they really weren't aware of any excesses or incorrect eating habits until they visited the doctor's office.

CJ's story isn't, unfortunately, unusual. It's like that of thousands and thousands of kids across America. Adolescent obesity has become an epidemic, but it's not up to the government or the schools to handle the problem. Handling obesity, and even preventing it in the first place, rests in the hands of two parties: first, it's the parents' job because they're the ones in charge of feeding their kids. Second, it's the responsibility of health-care practitioners — pediatricians, physician's assistants — to help educate the parents on what a healthy diet really is.

Obesity, the harmful excess of body fat, has become one of the most important health issues facing Americans in the twenty-first century because obese individuals tend to develop all the chronic diseases that are expensive to treat and remain elusive to cures — diseases like diabetes, osteoarthritis, and even cancer. It can become dangerously unhealthy to be classified as obese. But we're also faced with a very insidious problem: the media has sucked us into thinking something is "healthy" because the commercial says so. What the commercial touts as "healthy" is oftentimes anything but. Take your everyday variety of breakfast cereal — the ones that "kids like to eat." They are loaded with sugar or high fructose corn syrup to improve the taste, and even if the cereal is "fortified" with vitamins and minerals, the rest of the stuff in the food negates anything nutritious that may or may not be in the cereal.

How Did We Get Here?

The incidence of obesity in children is currently showing a steep upward curve compared to only a few decades ago. In the 1970s, the rate of childhood obesity was about 7 percent, and by 1999 it had increased to about 20 percent. According to *Webster's* definition of epidemic — "a phenomenon that is prevalent in the community and spreading rapidly among many individuals" — childhood obesity is now an epidemic. While there have been various studies that point to different causes of obesity, the simple fact is that weight gain, whether it is a little or a lot, is caused by an increase in food intake and a decrease in energy expenditure. To put it in the simplest of terms: if you eat more and exercise less, you're going to gain weight. If you eat a lot more than what you need and don't exercise or do anything to burn off the extra calories, then you're going to gain a lot of weight.

However, that simple definition does not encompass the very complex relationship we have with food. Food has become something other than simple nourishment to modern-day human beings. Some food makes us feel good — that's why it's called "comfort food." Some foods possess a cultural connection that is important to us. We see actors and actresses on TV eating and drinking every day, so we do the same. We snack. A lot. We give ourselves "treats" when we feel bad or to celebrate something good.

The very foundation of our culture, the family, has also seen changes in its relationship to food. Through the 1950s, there was someone in the home, usually the mother, to prepare food for the family. Setting out chips and soda for dinner was out of the question. As women started to venture more and more into the workforce, less time remained for food preparation.

Enter fast food. The industry advanced to meet the increasing demands of the growing number of two-income families with little time for food shopping and preparation. Coupled with that was the changing nature of how we lived. When more and more families moved out to the suburbs in the 1960s, the automobile became increasingly necessary, and fast-food joints popped up on every corner. Back then, they offered less expensive meals than could be cooked at home.

Other parts of the food industry jumped on the "convenience" bandwagon. Boxed food that could be made quickly crowded grocery-store shelves. The soft drink industry did not lag in its innovation of products: if athletes needed a refreshing drink, there was a "sports drink" that claimed to replenish water and electrolytes. Of course, the commercials didn't tell you that these same drinks came with a good dose of carbohydrates added to make them tastier. If a child was a picky eater, no problem; there was a delicious and nutritious liquid meal — along with plenty of sugar to make it tastier.

Then came the 1970s and 1980s, and we started to realize we had a problem. Doctors observed an increase in their patients' weight, and the first research articles trying to define the problem appeared. Then, we had an "aha" moment: we related the amount of fat accumulating in our bodies to the amount of fat we ingested. It made sense; if we are getting fat, it must be because we are consuming too much of it. And so began the "fat-free" revolution.

This first diet trend was all about decreasing the amount of fat in the diet. The food industry created and promoted foods that claimed

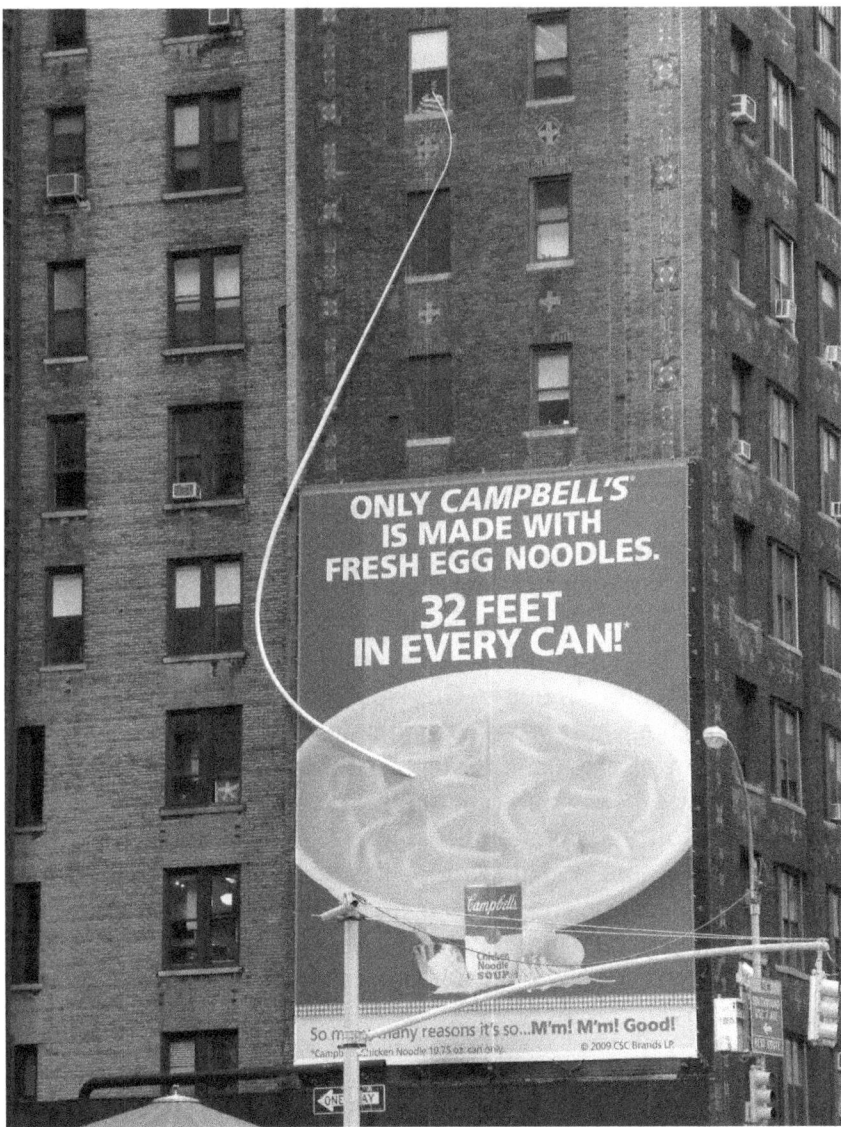

to be low in fat and, therefore, "good for you." However, despite all efforts to keep the amount of fat in our diets low, more than twenty years later, we were still not seeing a reversal of the obesity epidemic. Why? After being told to eliminate fat in our diets, we compensated by increasing the amount of carbohydrates. And thus created the next fad: low-carb diets.

People lost weight when they didn't eat bread or cereal or pasta, just like they did when they stopped eating fat. But in the 1990s our waistlines kept growing. Why? A low-carbohydrate diet is as out of balance as a low-fat diet. Carbohydrates are as necessary for healthy body function as fat or protein. The good kind of carbohydrates — complex carbs like whole grains, fruits, and veggies — not only taste good, they add essential nutrients like vitamins and minerals to our diet. Our bodies need them.

We are not moving in the right direction, obviously. When I ask kids, as part of my new-patient intake process, what they ate over the last couple of days, they name a number of visits to fast-food places and describe food choices that include fat-loaded, carbohydrate-drenched, sugar-added meals that would make our grandparents roll over in their graves. When I ask parents what they did for the weekend, they come up with the same description. If I ask kids what they like to eat, they never mention a family-cooked meal as they did in the past. When I was growing up, I remember asking my grandma to prepare my favorite meal. Not anymore! Now kids ask grandma to take them to a fast-food chain restaurant.

I don't know how else to put this — our lives are at stake here because our health is being compromised, daily, by the food we choose to put in our mouths. Our kids are not only missing out on good health, but when we allow others (like the advertising industry) to teach them what is good for them, and when we deprive them of the experience of eating homemade, quality meals, they are also missing out on traditions and memories. Rare is the day when a child comes home and declares, "It smells like dinner," because mom has a roast baking in the oven. If we don't change now, our kids are going to continue the trend with our grandkids, and we'll all witness the emergence of generations that have a shorter lifespan than ours.

Quality, Quantity, and Timing: A Healthy Way to Think about Eating

Professor Francisco Grande Covian, a Spanish doctor and professor, was an expert in nutrition. He was also a very wise man with a unique character and wit. On one occasion, a reporter who was looking for an easy answer to the obesity problem asked him, "Professor, what food makes us lose weight?"

He answered with his calm, deep voice, "The food you leave on your plate."

We gain weight because we eat too much, plain and simple. There is no single ingredient or nutrient responsible, but if we must find a culprit, the consumption of carbohydrates (sugars) in their various forms tends to be habit forming.

However, going on a diet is about as appealing to people as going to get a wisdom tooth pulled—and even that's a bad comparison because the trip to the dentist is only painful for a little while. Diets don't work. Getting upset about eating the wrong foods only seems to make you want to eat them more. There has to be a better solution to this problem!

In the preface, I talked about the need to go back to an old-fashioned form of eating—from scratch. Cooking that uses fresh foods, not something that comes from a box or from a can, goes a long way toward maintaining healthy weight. But there is more to it. Over the years, I have developed a way of thinking about food, a three-pronged approach that actually creates new food habits. This is the approach that I carry through this book, which culminates in the **Step Up Diet**. As will be made clear, there is a way to prevent and handle childhood obesity.

There is a way to enjoy food without having it get out of control, and it involves simply—with some discipline—paying attention to the quality of the food we eat (Quality), the amount we consume (Quantity), and when we eat (Timing). I've come to call it the QQT approach to healthy eating, and like any habit, once we train yourselves to ask the key QQT questions before we eat—anything—we'll retrain yourselves in no time. Once we get used to the new habits, life becomes easy again, and good health is just around the corner.

Throughout the book, I will present various aspects of the quality, quantity, and timing approach, so I am not going to explore them in-depth here. But the following general summary provides an introduction to the idea so that when I discuss any one aspect of QQT, you will know immediately what I'm talking about.

Quality

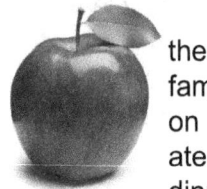

Economic shifts in the past few decades, including the move from the city to the suburbs, turned many families from reliance on one income to dependence on two incomes family, changing the way Americans ate. Because mom no longer was at home making dinner every night, the quality of what we have been putting into our mouths has suffered. I could go on and on about fast food—and I will in a bit—but let's just take a quick look at one of the enemies of quality food: prepared, processed foods. Once people no longer had the time to make dinner from scratch, we turned to prepared foods that, as advertised, were easy to fix and ready in minutes: macaroni and cheese, microwaved meals, even frozen "TV dinners"—all you had to do was pop them in the oven. Processed foods are advertised as "healthy," but they aren't. They're full of salt and sugar to make them taste good, and they are also full of other food additives like dye to make them look good.

The quality of our food has long suffered at the expense of convenience. Sometimes poor-quality food is cheaper, sometimes not. But one thing is certain: the quality of the food we eat affects the quality of our health. Convenience is based on getting something quickly, and Americans tend to want what they want *now*. Whenever we are asked to choose between quality and convenience, in our twenty-first-century world, we lean toward convenience. But I want you to stop and consider—at what cost?

What really is more convenient in the end? Is it spending less time and maybe less money on food? But what if that food makes us fat and unhealthy so that we spend more time than we should at the doctor's and far more money than we want on medication to handle the problems caused by poor-quality food?

That's the choice we face.

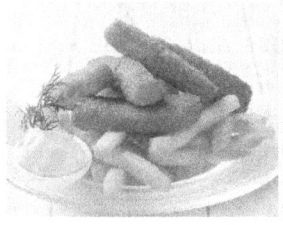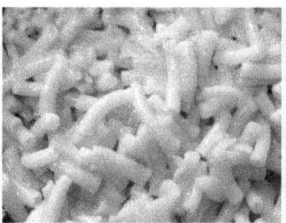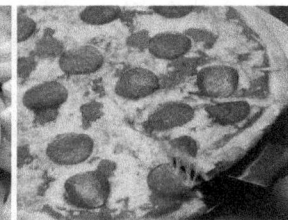

Quantity

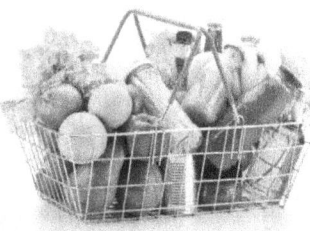

Quality is also being compromised by quantity — both the quantity of food and the quantity of food choices.

Visit any restaurant, and you're going to feel cheated if your plate isn't overflowing with food. We see commercials with plates heaped with food.

But it's not just the amount of food restaurants serve up. Think about when you sit down in front of the TV to watch a game or a movie, and mow through a bag of corn chips, a pint of salsa, or a liter of soda — that's simply too much food.

The problem is also compounded by the many choices we're given. From my point of view, it is a mistake to give children food choices. If they're hungry, put something fresh and/or homemade in front of them. Today, children have choices at school and choices at home. No wonder they always end up eating the same low-quality food.

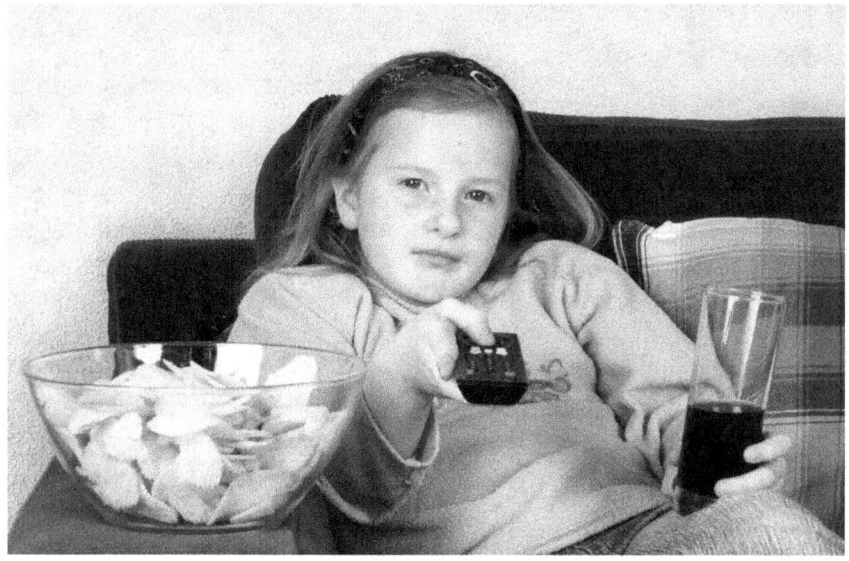

In my medical practice, I have treated adolescents who told me they ate pizza every day. They go home and eat snacks while watching TV then go out for fast food at dinner. They drink only soft drinks, some of which contain phosphates that promote calcium loss. This creates brittle bones at an early age. These kids complain to me of feeling so tired they cannot concentrate in school, and do not perform well when playing sports. I tell them, "You are what you eat — this is the truth."

My patients hear me repeating this advice ad nauseam: "No juice, no sodas, no chips, and no candy — allow these things only on special occasions." A few days ago, I was at the local grocery store when a six-year-old girl approached me and said, "Hello, Dr. Katalenas. Remember me? I saw you in your office yesterday." I assured her that I remembered her, though I couldn't think of her name. She went on to remind me that she was the girl who I instructed not to drink sodas or juice.

Her mother, close behind her, smiled and replied to her, "Oh honey, Dr. Katalenas says that to everybody."

It is true that I repeat myself when it comes to this important reminder. My older patients, after hearing the same song year after year, recite it to me each time I walk through the examining room door.

Timing

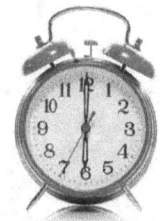

The third important component of a sound approach to good nutrition is timing. Meals and snacks should be scheduled. Period.

Ideally, children's mealtimes should be scheduled about four hours apart. If we time breakfast as nearly as possible to waking up and dinner as nearly as possible to bedtime, we can easily schedule lunch in the middle of the day and snack time between lunch and dinner. For most children, snack time should wait until after school; for toddlers, it should follow their afternoon nap.

A patient of mine asked me why I insist on giving kids just four meals a day and eliminating all other snacks. The answer is very simple: while some diet plans advocate eating several small meals throughout the day — some, up to eight — they are designed for adults who are already overweight and want to lose weight. Those plans offer a stepped-down approach; that is, they start decreasing the amount (quantity) of the meals first while maintaining a high frequency of meals, in order to make it easier for the person to engage.

My approach introduces timing right away; I think it is important to start training the body—and the brain—to go without food for a number of hours and to offer only good food (quality) without options. By following this schedule, the amount of food we consume during a whole day (quantity) will be automatically decreased. Because this book is geared to helping the whole family, I don't advise training a young person to eat too many meals or snacks. Otherwise, when the child becomes an adult, he or she will likely end up overeating and becoming obese.

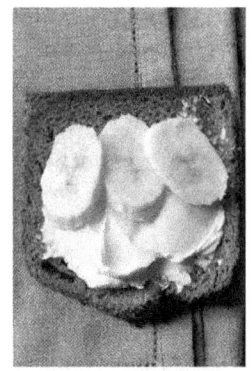

When setting up a meal plan for a family with small children, even if they are not obese, the goal is to provide good nutrition and to initiate good habits, training the body to go without food for three to four hours at a time. There is no animal species on earth that needs to be constantly eating or drinking as if connected to a calorie-producing umbilical cord. We should be able to go through the day without having food nearby. We don't need to keep food in the drawers at work or visit the refrigerator during every TV commercial break when we are at home. These are bad habits, ones that are causing our children to be overweight.

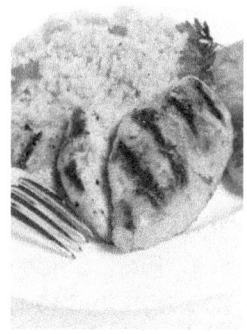

Taking Back Healthy Traditions

It's time to take back that which we have lost. Yes, bad habits are hard to break. I suggest starting now to always make food choices based on quality, quantity, and timing. This is especially true if you have young children in the family. They are going

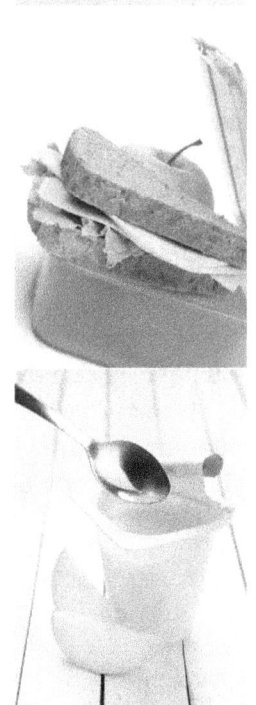

to learn their eating habits at home; they are going to learn primarily from their parents.

Food prepared outside of the home and packaged snacks are readily available, seemingly affordable and practical, but they are designed to make us eat more than we need. The way to alleviate the problems inherent in eating a lot of poor-quality food all the time is to put on that old stained apron, open up a cookbook (or watch one of the many cooking shows now on cable TV), and fire up the stovetop or oven. Cooking is an art. No, it isn't as convenient as opening a bag or stripping off some plastic wrap. But it can be a cheaper alternative to fast food or prepared food, and while it requires some clean up, think of it as a stress reliever at the end of the day.

The fight against obesity is going to require us to meet a most difficult challenge: to change our food habits and our lifestyle around eating. We can do it, and we must do it. Our children's lives depend on it.

Remember CJ? This is how he and his parents might use the QQT approach to prevent something none of them want — an obese child. First, adjustments need to be made, both to the number of meals offered to CJ and to the quality of the food he is offered. To begin with, breakfast need only be served to him once per day.

Second, his parents could replace his after-school snack of packaged foods with fresh fruits and milk sent from home. They can also eliminate any further snacking before dinner time while CJ spends that time playing (preferably outside) instead of eating. Since he will be hungry at dinner time, CJ will be more ready and willing to eat a balanced meal in the evenings. He will consume protein and carbohydrates in more reasonable proportions instead of eating only carbohydrate-loaded side dishes.

And finally, if dinnertime is moved a little bit closer to bedtime, his parents can avoid having to offer one more meal or snack.

It takes some planning, some discipline, and some effort on everyone's part, but the results will be noticeable. How do I know? CJ is my patient, and he is now no longer at risk of becoming obese.

How to Use This Book

This book is divided into three parts. Part 1 is geared toward helping you become aware of some of the food habits and choices you have taught to your children that are contributing to their expanding waistlines. It is not meant to make you feel guilty about what you've been feeding your child. Rather, I point out the problems so that you can fix them and move on to enjoying a healthier body and a happier life.

At the end of each chapter in part 1, I provide a list of "helpful tips" for overcoming the problems I present in that chapter (like those just below). I want to be very clear: this isn't a conventional diet book. It is not meant to grind you down with subtle, subliminal messages about how you should or shouldn't look, or feel about your body. It is meant to be nurturing, like a delicious bowl of homemade soup, so that you feel good about how you're treating your body.

Above all, this is a book about choices, and parts 2 and 3 offer practical suggestions on how to put the quality, quantity, and timing approach to work, culminating in the *Step Up Diet*. For if this solution to obesity is about anything, it's about making smart choices when it comes to food. I've said it before, and I'll say it thousands of more times while I'm still breathing—we are the ones who decide what food goes into our mouths. We are the ones who can be in control of what we eat so that we can maintain good health.

You will see how it can all come together, in a step-by-step fashion. You will get recipes, grocery lists, and menus to help you get started. But always remember this: nothing ever gets done immediately. Any job, if you think about it, requires that we do one thing, then another, then another. Changing our eating habits is no exception.

For now, the following list is your first taste of how QQT can be applied to everyday eating habits.

Helpful Tips

— Offer homemade food to the family as often as you possibly can. By cooking at home, the quality factor of the nutrition equation is being taken care of.

— To deal with time constraints, cook twice a week, keeping food in the refrigerator or freezer for the rest of the days.

— Make two trips to the grocery store per week. To prevent spoilage, buy only the ingredients needed for the food you are about to prepare.

— Schedule four meals a day: breakfast, lunch, after-school snack, and dinner. Since children eat lunch at school, either choose to send a homemade lunch or pay for a school lunch in hopes that the right choices will be made. In time, a child will apply the food habits learned at home to any situation where given a choice, such as at school or when visiting at friends' homes.

— Offer food only at mealtime — no short-order cooking or eating while watching TV. Mealtime should mean a family gathering around the table.

— Have a bowl of fresh fruit available and visible in the kitchen. When dealing with a teenager who can't wait until dinner, a piece of fresh fruit should be an option.

— Offer only water or milk to drink with meals and only water in between meals.

— Allow a child to eat as much as desired during mealtime. If a child is obese, use a smaller plate for serving and restrict seconds.

— Offer one main dish per meal, minimizing the amount of side dishes.

Every tip I offer in this book has been proven to work over and over by my patients in the twenty-five-plus years I have practiced medicine. They are all very kid-friendly; I know because my patients, the wonderful children I help to maintain in good health year after year, tell me so. And above all, I know that the Step Up Diet will help you because the many moms and dads who have used the program have found that it not only helps their kids, but also helps them gain control over their own poor eating habits, yet in a way that still allows them to enjoy good food.

That is what I want for you, so onward ho! Let's tackle this problem of obesity once and for all!

Part I

The Problem

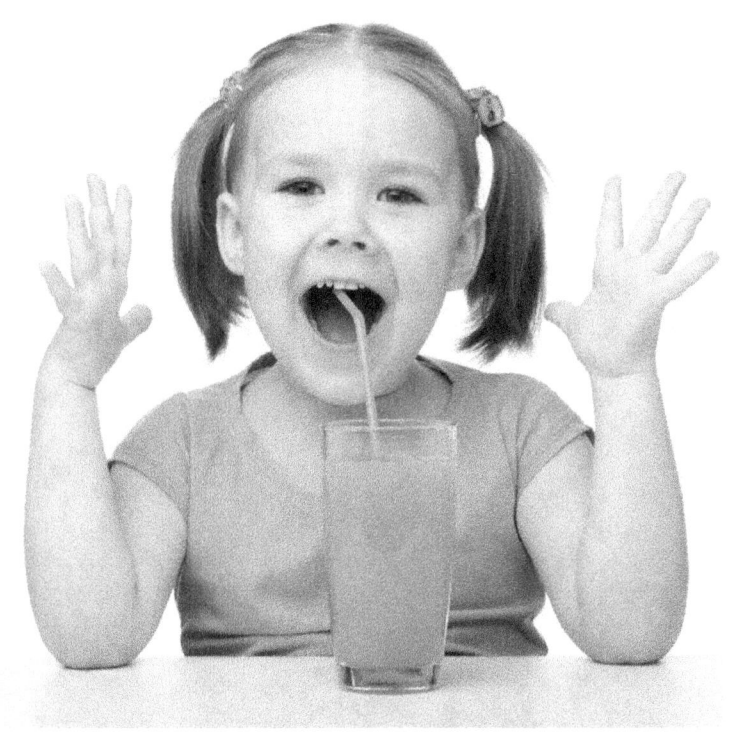

Chapter 1

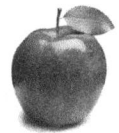 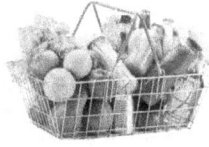 

The
Fruit Juice
Conspiracy

Sweeeeeet!!!

If I had to pinpoint one culprit, one thing that our kids eat too much of that causes them to gain too much weight, I would say sugar. Hands down.

Have you ever wondered why so many adult Americans have a sweet tooth? It all starts in childhood when we train our kids to drink sweet drinks when thirsty, and it continues with the fact that most of the prepared foods we consume contain sugar. All the commercial sauces in the supermarket, such as ketchup, mayonnaise, barbecue sauce, tartar sauce, and salad dressings contain added sugar. We don't even notice it because we are so accustomed to it.

Let's just take mayonnaise as an example. As an adolescent, I liked mayonnaise. A lot. I remember my years as a college student in Spain when I made sandwiches of just bread with mayonnaise when nothing else was available. When I came to the United States as a young woman, I found the taste of mayonnaise too sweet compared to what I was used to. For years, when I would visit Spain, I would return to my U.S. home with a couple of jars of the Spanish mayonnaise—with the tangy flavor I preferred. And much to the amusement of my friends, when they came to visit and asked what I wanted from Spain, I would ask for a jar of mayonnaise.

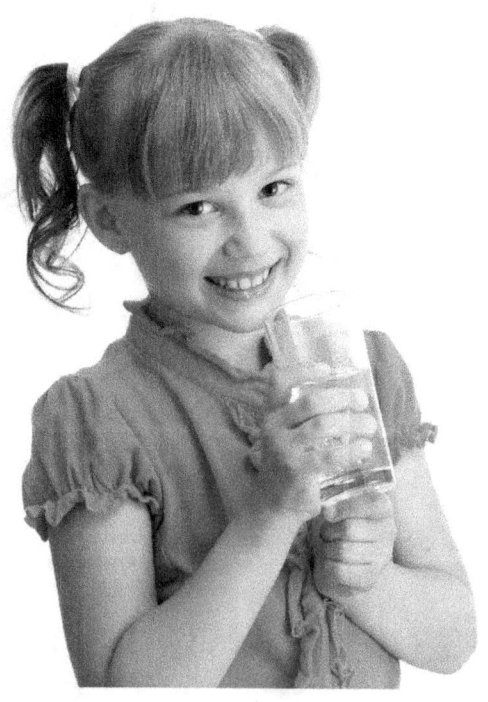

It took me a few years to get used to the taste of American mayonnaise, but I did. Now, twenty-five years later, I have to say I find Spanish mayonnaise too sharp, and I much prefer the American-made brands. My taste buds learned to like the sweeter condiment.

In the introduction, I talked about how much of our prepared food is loaded with sugar. Sugar is added to many foods to help preserve them and to make them more palatable. The most common additives are refined beet or cane sugar and high fructose corn syrup. They are added to sodas and other drinks to improve their taste.

But there's the heart of the problem. When our kids say they are thirsty, what do we give them? Not water, unfortunately. We give them juice. Or Gatorade. Or Kool-Aid. Colored drinks loaded with sugar.

We know sugar is bad. Drinking juice and eating sugary foods regularly predisposes children to dental decay. We know that. But what happens when we give children beverages with added sugars on a regular basis? We are training their taste buds to crave sweets, and by the time they are adolescents, they are not interested in drinking anything else.

I had one mother tell me that when someone observed her giving water to her toddler, the mother was scolded. She was told that children needed to be drinking juice. The mother was floored. When did water become "bad"? It never did. It's that our perception of what is "good" for our children changed because sugary drinks are what are advertised.

Water is cheap. Corporations make money on sweetened drinks that may contain added vitamins and minerals, but as I have already pointed out, the added nutrients are negated by the effects of the sugar on the body.

Sugar Addiction

Parents who consume sugary drinks on a regular basis relate to me how their "addiction" began when they were children when they were encouraged by *their* parents to drink flavored drinks. The habit is very difficult to reverse and is often passed down to the next generation.

Thomas, for example, is a ten-year-old boy who practices soccer twice a week and plays outside after school for an hour each day. Before and after exercise, his parents encourage him to drink fluids in the form of calorie-free flavored water because he prefers it to plain water. Along with his parents who drink sodas regularly, Thomas drinks sugar-free sodas with meals.

But the problem begins early. Mario is a two-year-old toddler who attends daycare where he plays outside every day, and he goes to the park in the afternoon with his mother. He never seems to have the need to drink. But his mother worries he is not getting enough fluids to maintain hydration, so she provides him with a sippy cup of watered-down juice to carry around throughout the day.

This is a very common situation. Parents are so afraid of dehydration that they create overhydration while cultivating in children at a very early age a dependence on sweet drinks. The problem actually is simple. Watered-down juice has a sweet taste, and it is going to be preferred over plain water. If Mario is offered watered-down juice, he is going to drink it even when he is not thirsty just because it tastes good, and he'll end up drinking more fluid than necessary. But that's not really the problem. For toddlers, juice is the equivalent of candy, and just as they will eat candy when not hungry, they will drink juice when not thirsty. If Mario is offered only water, on the other hand, he is going to drink it only when he is thirsty.

Our bodies regulate how much fluid we need by means of the thirst mechanism. When we need fluids, the body sends signals to the brain, and the sensation of thirst is felt. Water is the fluid our body needs when we are thirsty.

Some toddlers reach for the sippy cup when they are bored, in the car, or when upset. A new problem is then created: the association that the brain makes between stress and sweet-tasting drinks. As an adolescent, Mario will need to drink sodas on a regular basis. He has become addicted to sugar.

Sugary Drinks and Diabetes

Allowing our children to constantly drink something that is full of added sugar, fructose, or corn syrup has some pretty severe consequences on their bodies. When we drink juice, the sugar from the juice is absorbed rather quickly, creating a rise in blood sugar. When our blood sugar rises, it stimulates the pancreas to produce insulin to assimilate all that sugar into the cells. As fast as blood sugar goes up, it comes down.

What do people with diabetes do when suffering an episode of low blood sugar (hypoglycemia)? They drink juice! This results in the quick normalization of the blood sugar. Those of us who don't suffer from diabetes *don't* need to have rushes of blood sugar produced by drinking juice throughout the day. That is true for adults as well as for children.

The overriding issue here, though, is that the overstimulation of the pancreas could lead to insulin resistance and, later on, to diabetes. Take the toddler, Mario. As an adult, if he is genetically predisposed, he may develop diabetes.

That's right. Allowing your child to drink sugar-laden drinks could cause diabetes to occur. Diabetes is not something you want to wish on anyone, especially your children.

Somehow our body is ready to handle the natural sugars present in some foods. I am referring to the sugar present in fruits and vegetables, as they are mainly carbohydrates (sugars) in composition. Once we start extracting the natural sugars and offering them alone (as when we squeeze the juice out of the fruit), or worse when we start adding sugar to other foods, the pancreas suffers such a demand for insulin production that at some point it fails to keep up and the production of insulin is insufficient to meet the demand. The body now is unable to process carbohydrates, which are incapable of entering the cells (without insulin, or with too little insulin, the cell can't burn carbohydrates for energy production). Cells then start burning fat for energy production, and the amount of sugar in the blood starts to rise. We now have a situation called diabetes mellitus. The long-term effects of high sugar in the blood are very devastating and well known. The heart suffers, predisposing the individual to heart attacks. The blood vessels a become lined by atheroma, a lining of fat that makes the circulation more difficult and strokes more likely. The kidneys, the brain, the retina . . . diabetes affects the whole body. Once the diagnosis is made, there is no cure. There is treatment, but there is no known cure for diabetes.

If an adult with diabetes could turn the clock back, how far back would he go? My guess he would have to go all the way back to childhood, when he started learning eating habits that predisposed his body to its current situation.

When I talk to parents and families who have a genetic predisposition to diabetes, I explain to them how the clock can be turned back, and they now hold the key to making a difference in their children's lives by teaching them the right habits. But one of the main difficulties arises when it is realized that the entire family must

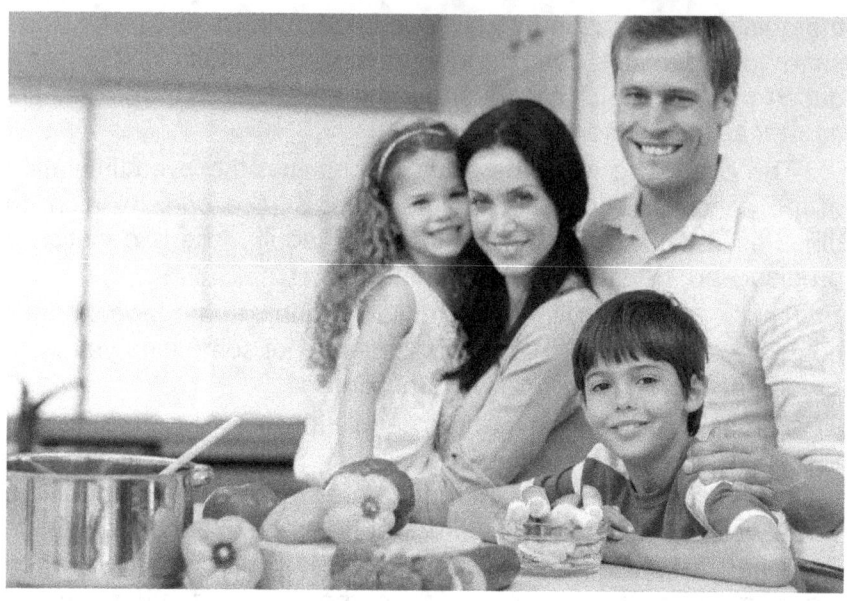

follow the right eating rules, not just the children. Therefore, just as the problem affects the whole family, the solution also must involve the whole family.

Sugar and Cholesterol

Diabetes is the most obvious disease that can arise from the consumption of too much sugar. However, too much sugar in our diets is also tied to elevated cholesterol.

We've all been warned about the problem of high cholesterol. Keep in mind there are two types of cholesterol: the good kind, HDL, and the bad kind, LDL and triglycerides. As adults, we need to be mindful always to lower the bad kind and increase the good kind. It keeps our hearts healthy.

Recent studies show that the consumption of added sugars in the diet contributes to an increase in LDL and triglycerides and a reduction in HDL. The mechanism by which this happens is not completely understood, but it seems to be mediated by fructose. Fructose is a naturally occurring sugar found most often in fruit. Fructose increases the liver's synthesis of triglycerides and other fats and interferes with the body's elimination of lipids—the fancy word for fat. In other words, sugar can create high cholesterol.

But wait, you say. High cholesterol is an adult problem. No, it is not. High cholesterol, an indicator and precursor of heart disease, is very much a problem in children, especially those who are obese or are headed that way.

Fruit Juice Isn't the Only Culprit

Tony is a fifteen-year-old athletic boy who has been instructed by his pediatrician to drink milk three times per day in order to increase the calcium intake for his growing bones. Tony is not a big fan of milk, but has promised to pay attention and make the effort.

At the time of his next visit to the doctor, he proudly reports he has been drinking three to four cups of chocolate milk every day in order to comply with the recommended calcium intake. In an effort to consume calcium, however, Tony is also ingesting a large amount of sugar with every cup of milk. Regular milk has about 11 grams of carbohydrates per cup, mainly from lactose (the sugar naturally present in milk). Chocolate milk, by contrast, has about 39 grams of sugar per cup.

Let's do the math: by drinking chocolate milk instead of regular milk, this child is taking in 84 extra grams of added sugar per day. When we 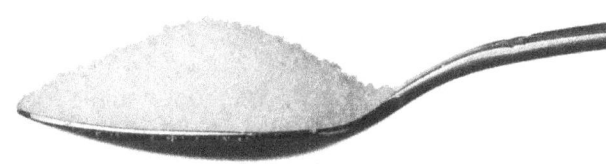 look at an entire month, it adds up to 2,250 grams or a total of 5.6 pounds of sugar. While the body is ready to manage the lactose naturally present in milk (assuming no lactose intolerance), the extra sugar will be accumulated in the form of fat unless the child engages in an incredible amount of exercise each day to burn it off.

Added sugars are not only present in beverages. Knowing our acquired preference for sweet-tasting food, manufacturers add more sugar to all kinds of products. For example, one unit of Activia fruit yogurt in the United States contains 19 grams of carbohy-drates; the same Activia brand of fruit yogurt in Spain contains only 8.7 grams. Bread in the United States typically includes sugar in its ingredients, while bread in other countries is usually made without added sugar. Not to mention salad dressing, ketchup, and other sauces: all are culprits in the list of sugar-laden foods.

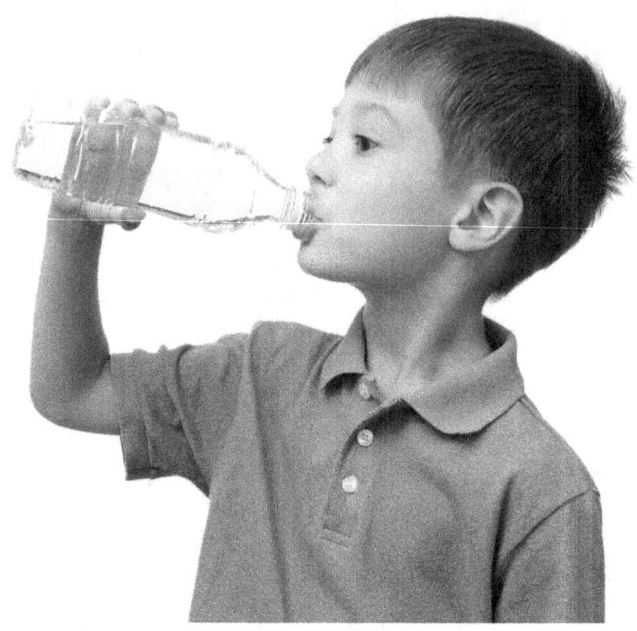

Training the Brain

The brain, which is responsible for all functions in the body, also has the ability to learn from its environment. So, in response to that environment, the brain directs the body in one manner or another, and it is in this way that habits are formed over time.

Because the brain learns what it is taught, we can always tweak the environment in a way that our brains learn more prudent habits, aiding in our impulse control and helping us maintain a healthier lifestyle. For example, research shows that meals that are low in carbohydrates produce a sensation that the brain reads as satiety for a long period of time. If we eat a big bowl of spaghetti for lunch, we immediately feel full and satisfied; our energy level goes up for a couple of hours, but it doesn't last long. In the middle of the afternoon, we start feeling sleepy and the stomach starts growling, signaling the need for more food. If, on the other hand, we consume a balanced meal with lower carbohydrates and more protein and fiber, the stomach takes a longer time to empty, and the brain learns not to crave food for a while longer.

Even if a child is given a glass of sweet-tasting juice only at times when he or she is thirsty, the brain learns to associate thirst with needing something sweet, and in time, the child is going to refuse any other fluids to quench a thirst. When a patient with dehydration arrives at the emergency room, the doctor is not likely to provide juice or any sweet fluid; oral rehydration solutions are not sweet—they are salty. And when the dehydration is severe enough to require intravenous fluids, what does the doctor administer? It is normal saline solution, which is just water and salt, without any sugar at all.

I have said this before, but it is so important I am saying it again. A child who is regularly given juice instead of water becomes an adolescent who will reach for a soft drink when thirsty, and an adult who will have a very hard time breaking a habit that may contribute to obesity, diabetes, or cardiovascular disease. Therefore, we must drop the fruit juice and reach for water if and when we are thirsty.

It comes down to a quantity and quality issue. If we acquire the habit of eating or drinking every hour, even if the amount of food or fluid ingested is small, the brain learns to expect a certain level of distension in the stomach, which it translates into a feeling of satiety. Therefore, when the stomach is empty for a short time, it initiates signals of discomfort (hunger) that prompt the person to seek food. This eventually creates the habit of overeating. The process is more involved than this, of course, and there are other hormonal factors that influence this signaling mechanism, but the sensation of hunger or feeling full comes from the brain, and thus is, in part, subject to training.

I could learn to like not-so-sweet Spanish mayonnaise again if I ate it all the time. Children can learn to drink water when they are thirsty if that is all that they are offered. Bodies get thirsty and eventually the body will drink whatever it is offered if it's thirsty enough.

Sugar and Picky Eaters

Yet another negative effect of children's habitual juice drinking is the depressive influence on appetite. A picky eater who drinks juice throughout the day is acquiring a number of empty calories that will decrease an already skimpy appetite and result in eating even less food. When dealing with a picky eater, we must eliminate soft drinks, fruit juices, and other flavored drinks, making sure only milk is served with their meals and water in between meals.

Food should be offered strictly at scheduled mealtimes; as they say, it's all about timing. By providing a meal every three to four hours, we make sure the child is hungry when he or she sits at the table. Hunger is the first requirement to encourage eating, just as thirst is the first requirement to motivate drinking. And as for "liquid meals," these kinds of drinks are ideal under certain circumstances, such as when a child is sick and unable to tolerate food. But for a healthy child who is just a picky eater, or who may even be using mealtime as an opportunity to challenge a parent's rules, liquid meals give the wrong message, and they can't be maintained in the long run. Eventually, the child is going to have to learn to eat normal food. Providing a liquid meal option doesn't make it any easier. When planning meals for a picky eater, we may take likes and dislikes into consideration only to a certain point. After all, we want to create and teach the variety rule that will carry into adulthood. A preferred food may be offered as the reward for first eating something less desirable.

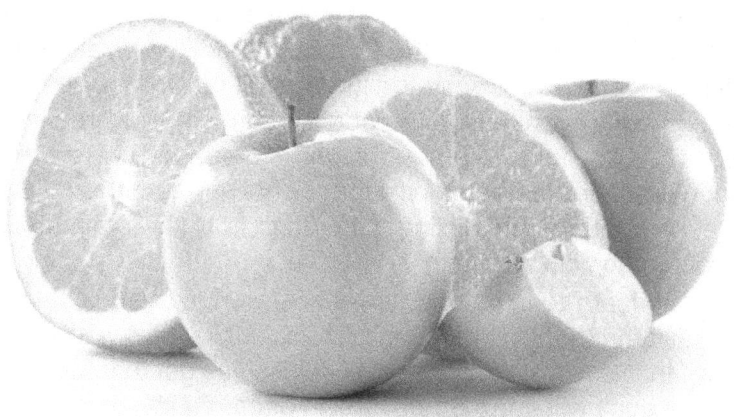

I also have to interject here a quick discussion on the difference between fruit and fruit juice. Some experts declare there is no difference between added sugars and naturally occurring sugars because, after all, sugar is sugar, right? *Wrong!* Naturally occurring sugars—for example, the sugars in a piece of fruit—exert their nutritional value when the *whole* fruit is consumed. While the fruit has natural sugars, it also contains fiber, which slows down the absorption of the natural sugars, and the final effect is beneficial. So, while some parents believe fruit juices are a good choice for kids, and they even count a glass of fruit juice as a serving of fruit, *an orange* and *the juice from an orange* are not the same thing. Even if squeezed at home with a juicer, juice is just water and sugar. Yes, it is "natural," but it doesn't compare to eating the whole fruit, which imparts the vitamins and fiber that contain the nutritional value and help with digestion.

Applying QQT

The American Heart Association (AHA) is asking for a reduction in the consumption of soft drinks and other sweetened beverages in an attempt to reduce the epidemic of obesity, which impacts heart disease. A recent report states that the average person in the United States consumes about 111 grams (22.2 teaspoons, or 335 calories) of discretionary sugar per day. The AHA proposed a reduction to 30 grams (6 teaspoons, or 100 calories) of added sugar for women and 45 grams (9 teaspoons, or 150 calories) for men. While the American Sugar Association and the American Beverage Association deny the allegations, the authors of this report allege that soft drink consumption is directly related to increased body weight.

Let's revisit some of the children I talked about earlier in this chapter. The easy solution for Tony, the kid who drank chocolate milk, is to drink plain milk with no added sugar. He just has to teach his taste buds to like milk. It can be done. Our taste buds learn what we teach them to like, just as I learned to like sweeter American mayonnaise. This explains, for example, why Mexican children can tolerate very hot, spicy food from an early age.

A good solution for Thomas' family would be to substitute water for the sugar-free drinks when he plays sports as well as with his meals. Sugar-free drinks may be calorie-free but they are not harm-free.

We still don't know what kind of effects artificial sweeteners may have when consumed over many years, and we do know that such drinks contain colorants and other chemicals that add no nutrients and can be difficult for the developing body to handle.

The solution for the toddler, Mario, is as simple as leaving the sippy cup at home and offering the child plain water when the environmental circumstances require some fluid intake. If he refuses the water, it only means that he is not thirsty and that he doesn't need a drink.

Helpful Tips

— Eliminate any flavored drinks, such as juice or flavored water, from the home. They have no nutritional value and lead to bad habits.

— Beverages with added sugar teach the brain to crave sweets and, in children, may mark the initial pathway to obesity, insulin resistance, and diabetes.

— Chocolate milk is not a good alternative to regular milk because it includes too much added sugar.

— Fruit juices should be consumed in moderation; they are not nutritionally equivalent to the whole fruit.

— While we cannot avoid all added sugar, which is present in so many foods, we can try to avoid the main sources. For children, this advice translates into offering only water or milk to drink.

— Learn to read labels to identify hidden added sugar.

— If thirsty between meals, drink only water.

— Parents hold the key to their children's future health. Eating habits are learned primarily at home, not at school. Childhood offers an optimal window for learning good eating behavior.

Chapter 2

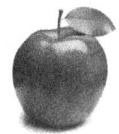 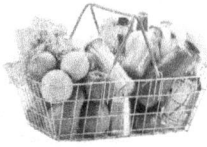 

The Culture
of Snacking

We Americans love our snacks. Entire grocery aisles are devoted to a myriad of chips, crackers, cookies, popcorn, and more. If it can be deep-fried or baked, it's going to be turned into a snack.

By definition, a snack is any food—healthy or not—that a person eats between meals. It's the easy stuff we reach for because we're hungry, or we're bored, or we need something to "pick us up."

Most of us realize that snacking isn't usually the healthiest way to approach food, but we all do it. It's comfort food, and I'm as guilty as anyone. This past summer my husband and I celebrated our twenty-fifth wedding anniversary with a trip to the Baltic countries. Since we go to Spain every summer, we decided to join a tour that departed from Madrid for one week of fun with thirty-four other Spaniards. We flew from Madrid to Vilnius, the capital of Lithuania, and from there we started a bus tour north, visiting different cities in Lithuania, Latvia, and Estonia. It was a wonderful trip. I learned much about the cultures of the Baltic region. Little did I know I would receive a lesson about my own culture, or rather about the blended culture of my life, my Spanish-American heritage.

The trip was very well scheduled, with bus stops every two hours for sightseeing or for a bathroom break at some highway service area. In other words, we never went more than two hours without getting off the bus. I started to observe my fellow travel mates as the days passed, and I noticed their behavior and how it differed from ours. One day, the tour guide was walking down the aisle of the bus and stopped at my husband's seat. The guide looked around at the little table in front of us and said, "Boy, you have a snack store here."

Looking at the other people, I realized we were the only ones with food in front of us. My husband had his bottle of tea on the table, and I had my water. We also had various little bags of nuts, pastries, and candy scattered over the fold-out tray table. Everyone else's tray table was up.

This prompted me to analyze our behavior. I found it interesting that I was so attached to my snacks since at home I make such a point of never eating between meals. Why was I compelled to change my behavior while on vacation? I came to the realization that since I was out of my regular environment and off my normal schedule, I felt the need to have food within reach because I feared I wouldn't have access to food at all. It was an emotional issue. Everyone, including me and my family, has emotional associations

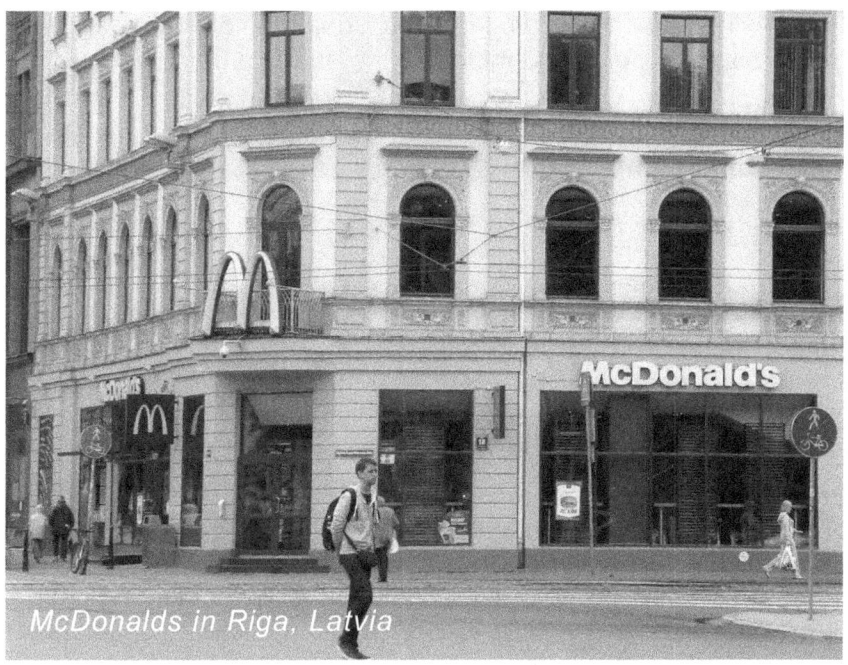

McDonalds in Riga, Latvia

with food. We each perceive food in a different way, depending on our upbringing and genetic makeup.

But none of that made me feel better. I knew better. I was aware of my invalid assumption, but that didn't stop me from buying snacks at our regularly scheduled stops. I even had my drink within reach at all times—something that I counsel others not to do.

What did my fellow Spaniards do? I can tell you, they did not eat or drink while in the bus. They did not have any food visible anywhere near them. When we had our scheduled stops, that's when they reached for their water or a cup of coffee. Most of them, however, just walked around, stretching their legs. We—Americans—were the only ones buying and eating food in between meals, and we were the only ones carrying a drink all the time. (It wasn't even that hot. It was June and the temperatures varied between fifty to seventy degrees. We weren't suffering from heat exhaustion, and we were never in danger of dehydration.)

This is not to say that our fellow travelers did not eat. They had a good appetite for quality food, and they were quick to criticize a few poor choices offered during the tour. But they reserved their appetite for mealtime. We had breakfast at the hotel every morning, and we had lunch and dinner at scheduled times. Some of them had a cup of coffee in the middle of the afternoon, but that was it.

It was an eye-opening experience for me and a humble reminder that, no matter where we are, we are a product of our culture and we tend to do what our culture teaches us to do, even when we know better.

The Problem with Snacks

This experience made me start to really pay attention to the problem of snacking in our diets. When I teach people the QQT program, I stress eating as the Spaniards do—at meals. That's the "timing" aspect of healthy eating: you eat every four hours. Then there are the quantity and quality issues. Have one healthy snack in the middle of the afternoon like an apple or some carrot sticks so that you don't feel overly hungry but have an appetite for dinner. If you're eating a healthy, balanced meal at mealtimes, you shouldn't feel overly hungry in between meals.

But perhaps hunger doesn't have as much to do with snacks as something else. In chapter 1, I talked about training your brain to not expect sweet drinks all the time. The same holds true for snacking. If we eat constantly, then we're training our brains to expect to feel a certain sense of fullness through the day. The "need" to keep a certain distension of the stomach and the intolerance to feeling hungry for a prolonged time is what makes snack food a comfort food. Snacks are usually not unnecessary from a nutrition standpoint, but are craved because they provide us with a comforting sensation.

Our culture of snacking, or food-for-comfort, extends to other aspects of our lives and no one is immune. I often attend medical conferences. These meetings go on all day long for one to five days. They usually start at 8:00 a.m. and end at 5:00 p.m. During all those long hours we are sitting, listening, learning, and asking questions. Breakfast is often served at 7:30 a.m., and food is allowed into the meeting rooms. The conferences are usually held in the ballroom of a big hotel, with hundreds of doctors attending.

We have fifteen-minute breaks every two hours and a one-hour break for lunch. The food is usually catered by the hotel, and typically it is healthy and balanced. That's not the problem. The problem is that during the breaks, snacks and drinks are served. There are

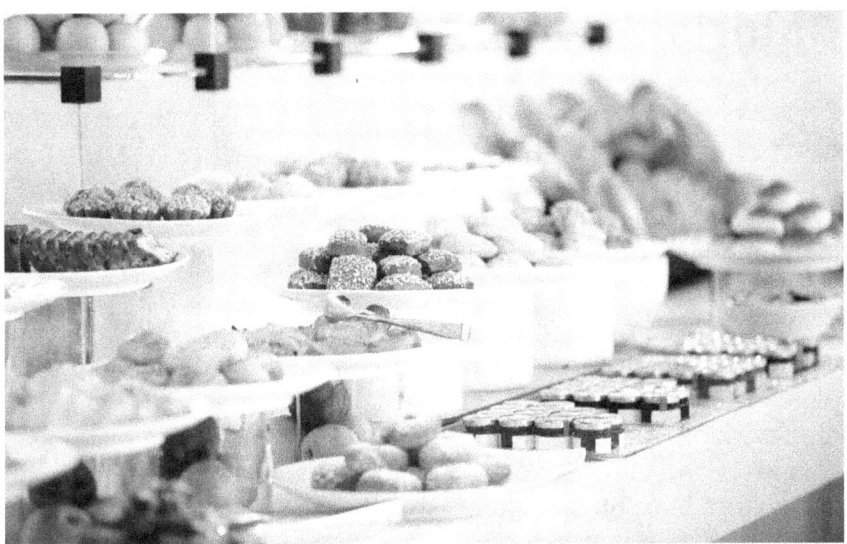

also dishes with hard candy at the tables and decanters with water. Needless to say, we spend the whole day eating.

The food provided during the breaks is superfluous; there's nothing we really need. We have been fed well just a few hours before, whether for breakfast or for lunch; nevertheless, we all gather around the snack tables full of pastries, sweet breads, and cookies—all of them quite tasty. There may be some fruit set out, and some of us hardier souls try to eat that. So we eat our snacks during the break, and then *we keep going* by bringing some of the snacks into the meeting room. Basically, we keep eating right up until dinner.

Clearly, none of the food provided during those breaks is good for us. But we are often mentally tired, and our bodies may feel sore from sitting too long. We could all use a massage, or a walk around the garden for some fresh air, or a bit of relaxation, like listening to some music or just stretching out on a comfortable sofa. But we eat. And eat. All that eating actually makes us feel more tired at the end of the day; however, the tradition is to eat. Why do we do it? Well, for one, it is there. Our feelings of tiredness get translated into hunger, and we eat because the food is in front of us. It is similar to the reaction we have in front of a dinner buffet, faced with the attraction of the colorful, delicious-looking food. The sensory input to our brains gets tangled with the awareness that we already paid for the all-you-can-eat menu, and we overeat.

Calorie Counting

Anyone who has ever tried to "diet" is familiar with the idea of calorie counting. Calories are simply the way that we measure how much energy a particular amount of food can produce. If we eat too much, we have taken in too many calories. Our bodies (some more than others) are programmed to store that excess energy capacity for emergency situations.

When it comes to children, I don't advise calorie counting. While it is simple logic that eating more food, therefore ingesting more calories, leads to an increase in body mass, the variables are so wide that it is not helpful or practical to spend time counting calories. For example, we all know plenty of kids who eat a lot, yet are able to burn off enough of what they eat to maintain a normal weight, and others who tend to accumulate weight even when they don't consume as much.

In theory, the daily calorie recommendation for a three-year-old is about 1,650, whereas an eight-year-old needs about 1,710 calories per day. A sixteen-year-old male who is engaged in light activity is recommended to consume approximately 2,549 calories each day, but a moderately active twenty-six-year-old female should consume about 2,212 calories per day and a reasonably active thirty-two-year-old male, about 3,500 calories per day. These are just statistical averages, and obviously the recommended numbers are too exact to be accomplished. My preference, therefore, is to concentrate more on the quality and the quantity of the food we take in, and this is where snacking becomes a real problem.

An eight-year-old girl, Jennifer, is identified by the school nurse as having an obesity problem. She is in the 95th percentile for weight and height for her age. She tends to eat seconds at the dinner table, and she drinks soda or chocolate milk with her meals and with her snacks. But it's the snacks where the calories really pile up.

In an effort to curb any further weight gain, her parents decide to restrict calories. When they try to calculate the number of calories Jennifer is consuming, they are surprised to find she is taking in about 1,800 calories per day. But is this number accurate? After all, this little girl eats like most other little girls in the United States. She eats lunch at school, and nobody (other than the girl herself) can say for sure how much she eats there. Does she go for seconds? Does she have access to side dishes, canned fruit, or granola bars as part of her lunch? (Granola bars are touted as "healthy" because they often contain whole grains, nuts, and seeds. That's all good stuff, but they are also loaded with sugar.)

Her parents also admit they had difficulty measuring the amount of calories in her after-school snack since the food is generally offered to kids without restriction, especially when it comes to the amount of juice they consume. The after-school program explains to parents that the children are given unlimited access to juice in order to prevent dehydration. Another gray area is the amount of calories the girl ingests at home prior to dinner. Jennifer is usually in her room playing or watching television, and she makes trips to the pantry as she feels the need.

The bottom line is that the amount of calories Jennifer's parents calculated may not be real. Even if the calorie count is reliable, knowing the number is not a solution in and of itself. Her parents still have to get more involved since the reality of her being over-weight requires some intervention.

Applying QQT

It is important to realize that even eliminating just a small amount of calories per day from a child's diet can make a significant differ-ence in achieving and maintaining a healthy weight. For example, knowing that a pound of fat contains approximately 3,500 calories, eating one cookie (60 calories) every day could mean an increase in weight by half a pound each month, and ultimately by six pounds in a year, and twenty-seven pounds over ten years. Conversely, by eliminating those few empty calories (calories that come from most snack food that are loaded with sugar and other unhealthy ingredients), we can reverse the equation and start losing pounds.

This example is for purposes of illustration only. Our bodies do not react to energy intake and expenditure in a concisely mathe-matical way; however, if we ingest calories above what we expend, we are going to accumulate weight. By the same principle, to lose weight, we have to restrict calorie intake and expend more energy.

In the case of Jennifer, a better approach to healthy eating would be to limit the opportunities (times and places) she has access to food. This would mean eliminating the many snacks. On top of that, it is important to change the quality of the food she is offered—water instead of juice; home-prepared foods at mealtime, from-scratch meals as often as possible. She can then be allowed to eat as much as her growing body needs without taking in too many calories.

According to the National Health and Nutrition Examination Survey (NHANES), young Americans ingest an excess of 370 calories per day. This is a direct correlation to the increase in overweight and obese children over the last thirty years. Children have an amazing ability to learn as they grow. Part of that capacity should be applied to learning healthy habits in order to achieve a healthier way of life.

By now we should have a clear idea about what we are doing wrong when it comes to the eating habits of our own family. I'm the first to admit that it takes a great deal of restraint and willpower to avoid the temptation to eat snacks. It all boils down to the quality-quantity-timing equation. If we keep those three words in mind always when we reach for food, healthy eating becomes a whole lot easier.

Don't be afraid, and be honest with yourself. Feeding our bodies is a primary need for all beings; when food is scarce, it becomes a major focus. But most of us face the opposite problem: we are presented with too much of it, and we must learn to manage our consumption before the excess destroys our own health.

Helpful Tips

— Calorie counting is an imperfect method of intervention when it comes to weight control in children.
— Different children have different needs, depending on their age and size and the amount of exercise in which they are involved.
— Concentrate on the type of food the child is offered and on how many times per day she or he is offered food.
— Parents have a say in the quality of the food their children are given at school and in after-school programs. If necessary, parents can provide their own fresh fruit, cheese, or milk to be kept on the premises and given to their child on a schedule.
— Some parents are afraid their child is going to be singled out if he or she eats differently from others. Think about the long-lasting consequences of allowing them to do "what everybody else is doing"— chronic disease and pain as an adult. They can be singled out now or later; it is up to us as parents.

Chapter 3

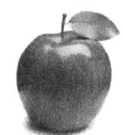 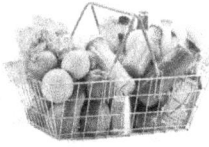 

There's a
Reason Why
It's Called a Treat

When my kids were small, we had a friend who would spend a few weeks at our home every summer. She is a lovely person, and for a long time I was puzzled why she was obese.

At mealtime, she always ate rather small amounts, so small that I sometimes felt bad about my cooking. In fact, she didn't seem to overeat in front of us. She assured me she always ate very little, and she was baffled why she continued to gain weight.

One day she pulled a small box of chocolates out of her purse and my youngest son, who was about six years old, took the only piece of chocolate out of the box and ate it. I scolded him because he didn't ask permission and had acted rudely. I pointed out he had taken the last piece in the box, leaving our friend with no more candy. She assured me not to worry and to leave the child alone, since she considered there was no reason to apologize.

At that point, everything became clear. She told me that she had plenty more chocolates around. She went to her car and brought out several similar boxes and offered them to my son, in an attempt to make him feel better after my scolding. To my surprise, she then went to her room and brought out an even bigger variety of candy and chocolates. I then understood a lot more about her relationship with food.

Kids and adults need to eat sweets every once in a while. You can't expect anybody to go through childhood without enjoying a cookie or a piece of cake as a treat. But the key word here is "treat." Food gives pleasure—like ice cream on a hot summer's day that you give your child because he or she was playing outside all day long. But treats should be reserved for special occasions like birthdays or other holidays. They are not meant for everyday consumption. Remember the cookie at 60 calories a day? Those calories add up fast.

Above all, the treats you give your children—and yourself—should be made at home. Desserts and pastries sold at stores contain a lot more sugar than they should, along with other chemicals and oils of poor quality. And let's face it—a cookie from scratch always tastes better than a store-bought one. If treats are for special occasions, make it truly special by making it yourself!

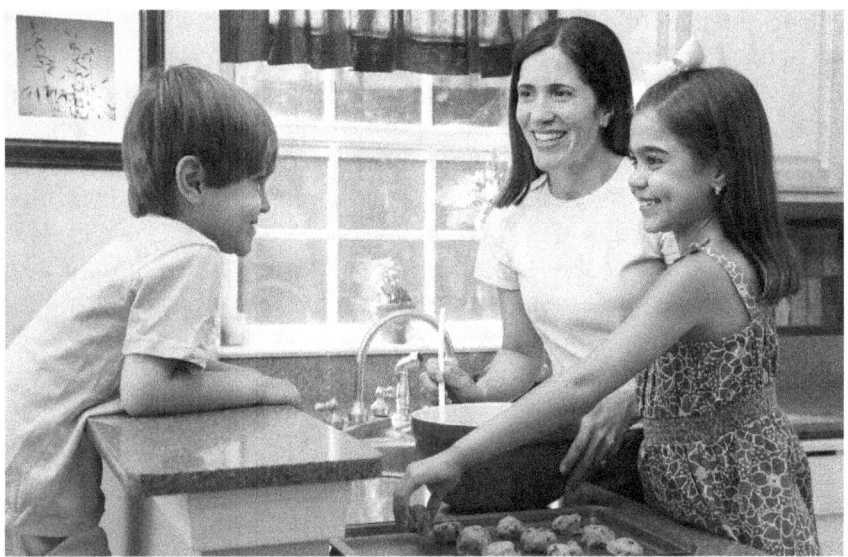

Treats Are Not Comforting

Last Christmas, there was an advertisement for a doll that would cry and need a Band-aid. That's all well and good, but the problem was, the doll asked for a popsicle—and there was a plastic one that the doll could then "eat."

This points to an effect that that we all know: the artificially created correlation between food and emotion. In other words, "comfort eating." Emanating from parents' desire to provide for their children, it starts early in life and continues throughout childhood. A toddler who is encountering a frustration during the day or is about to have a temper tantrum is given a bite to eat or a sip of juice producing a powerful calming sensation. The comforting effects in the brain from the splash of sweetness are great. Dr. Robert Pretlow studied the causes and consequences of "comfort eating" in adolescents who eat when stressed, angry, or lonely. He pointed to visible changes in the brain that are induced by this behavior; there is something in our brains called a dopamine pathway that leads to the release of endorphins. When we eat comfort food, those endorphins are triggered, and the subsequent soothing outcome has been well documented. What starts from a well-intentioned, gentle behavior becomes an ingrained, potentially harmful habit to which the brain is still prone into adulthood.

To put it bluntly, treats should not be something you give a child to help calm him or her down. Kisses and comforting words are calorie-free and do far more to calm a sobbing child—whether girl or boy—than a sugar-laden treat that might bring only temporary relief. Giving a child a treat because he or she is hurt also sends the message that something sweet is comforting. But, as we have seen, this message is one we have to unlearn. We need to train ourselves to find viable substitutes for all those treats. It may take some ingenuity, and it may not be as easy and fast as reaching for a cookie or a piece of candy.

The Difference between Fun and Fanatic

There are many ways to look at substitution for a treat. The kind of substitution I'm talking about is to give your kid a really neat pencil or a book instead of an ice-cream cone or some equally sugar-laden food. That is, use distraction in a way that doesn't involve food.

But I want to caution you here. Substitution does not mean that you make a sweet treat out of "alternatives" to the real thing. A friend of mine gave me the recipe for a cake she made for her daughter's birthday. She was so proud of this mixture she put together herself that I didn't have the heart to share with her my concerns. Since she is a very good cook and concerned about sugar added to food, she decided to make a cake using artificial sweeteners, some kind of simulated chocolate powder she found at a health food store, and simulated butter. All in an attempt to avoid the real sugar, chocolate, and butter she wanted to spare her daughter.

Here is my message. Nobody gains weight from eating their own birthday cake. Why? Because birthdays happen only once a year! That occasion calls for a treat, and to make my point loud and clear, I want to share a favorite recipe for a homemade dessert that is both easy and fast. Most of all, it is delicious and not too sweet. Ready?

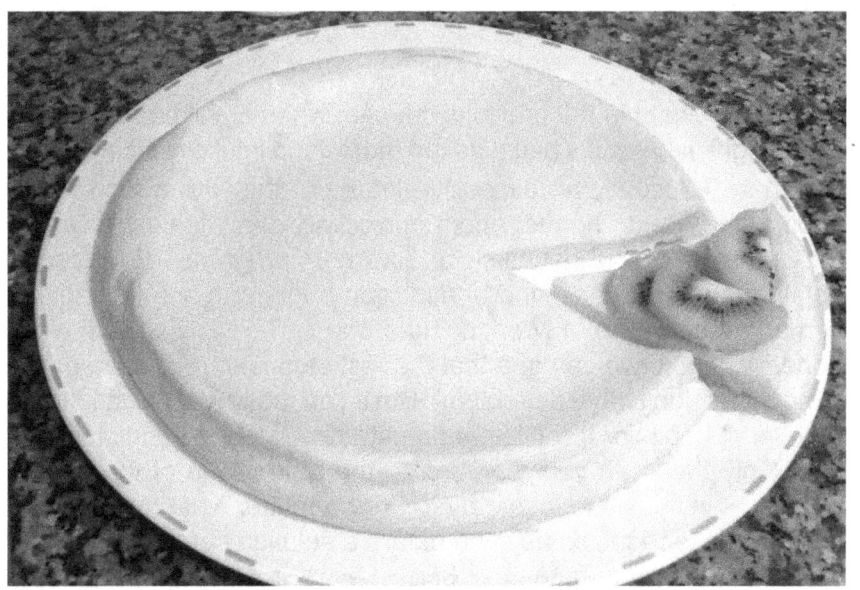

LEMON CUSTARD DESSERT

Ingredients
2 lemon yogurts*
2 containers flour
2 containers sugar
4 containers milk
2 eggs
5 tablespoons butter
ground lemon peel

* Note: Keep the yogurt containers because you need them to measure the other ingredients.

Preparation
Mix all the ingredients using a hand blender or food processor to make it smooth. Pour into a round oven-safe dish, about 8–9 inches in diameter and cook at 430 degrees for 45 minutes.

If you have company for dinner and you want to make it into individual dessert portions, bake it in a 13 X 9 inch rectangular dish. After it is cooked, allow it to cool off, turn it over, and cut it into individual portions. Place a blueberry or half of a strawberry on top of each portion and sprinkle each one with some powdered sugar.

Applying QQT

As I stressed in the previous chapter, when a child or an adult is overweight, it happens because too much food intake is taking place.

There is usually an excessive intake of the wrong food at the wrong time. Being honest about our quality-quantity-timing can be the start of a whole new life. In fact, most programs dedicated to helping those with any kind of addiction begin with a self-examination and recognition of wrongdoing. Food can be addictive. If we're honest about it, we can see that the first step is to recognize denial (who me? I don't have a problem). But if you really want to start living an overall healthier lifestyle, you must acknowledge denial for what it is. Only then can you move on to the recognition of the deeper problem—in this case, overeating. For no matter what the problem, it has to be recognized as such before a solution can be applied.

In this chapter, instead of giving you helpful tips, I'm going to have us take another look at my friend's situation, the one eating (too much) chocolate candy, and apply the quality-quantity-timing logic to her situation, but in steps that make it more manageable. As you'll see, QQT is holistic, and thus it can be approached from any of three angles.

Step 1 — Timing

After my friend admits the problem, the first step would be to work on timing. Since it is more difficult to apply all three steps at the same time, creating a schedule of meals first helps cut down on the amount of food (quantity) without much effort. She can also look forward to mealtime, knowing she can still eat what she likes when the next meal arrives.

She should first practice having four meals a day, separated by three to four hours, and need not worry at this point whether those meals contain the right type of food (or not) or the right amount (or not).

She should do just this step for about two weeks. Why? By allowing 3–4 hours in between meals, she will become accustomed to the sensation of hunger without reaching for food immediately, the first step in controlling her bad habit.

Step 2 — Quality

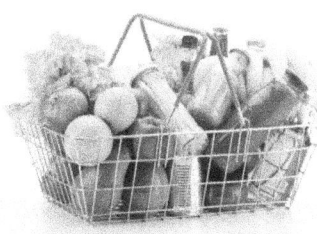

The second step could be working on the quality of the food. For the next three weeks, she should try very hard to not only keep the schedule of meals (four a day), but make a menu of nutritious food, like the meals described at the end of this book. She can eat as much as she wants of all the quality food she prepares. Why? By being stricter about the what she eats, or the quality of the food, she is also working on the amount she eats. We naturally tend to eat more of foods that are very attractive to us, which includes sweets and snacks, and we tend to eat less of a real meal.

Included in the quality of the food is the quality of the drinks she consumes. She should be drinking only water or milk (definitely no soda pop, fruit juices, or chocolate milk).

Step 3 — Quantity

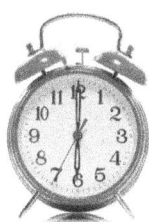

By going through the prior two steps, she may already be eating the right amount of food. But it would be worth the time to spend another two weeks applying what's she's already put in place, the meal schedule and the meal plan, with the final step being to work on not serving herself seconds and not using large plates. Because we tend to fill our plates full, large plates potentially mean too much food.

Once she has her QQT program in place, then she can give herself a treat—one piece of chocolate or one cookie, not a whole box.

This three-step plan can be followed by anyone—child or adult. One factor to take into account is that nothing happens overnight. The plan I just outlined takes seven weeks to complete. But it can take that long—and sometimes longer, much longer—to do something as difficult as changing long-established eating habits. But change them we must if we're going to give our children the gift of a long and healthy life.

Chapter 4

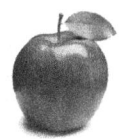 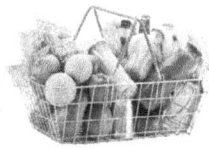 

Macaroni and Cheese, Pizza, and Other Fast-Food Blunders

I am not going to blast my fury at the fast-food industry, blaming them for all the bad in our diet. The responsibility resides in the individual, and when the individual is a minor, it falls directly into the parent(s). It's as simple as that.

I believe the fast-food industry in this country followed a niche of opportunity, in response to the changes in society created by families' needs to have more flexibility and convenience when it comes to their food choices. Just like any other industry, this one saw a need and proceeded to fill it by creating fast, affordable food that is available anywhere at all times.

Fast-food restaurants became icons of American culture that we exported very successfully to other countries. I feel the emotion inside when I spot the Golden Arches in a faraway land, I must confess. They are a symbol of American enterprise and success and McDonald's creates thousands of jobs and economic opportunities, we must not forget.

I can imagine that the fast-food industry will change, but only when society and individuals change. Once parents improve their eating habits, a natural consequence would be to that they would desire or expect the same quality when they eat out and will refuse to settle for less. As a result, restaurants would have to offer only the best ingredients in smaller amounts, even if that translates into higher costs.

Economic decision making indirectly affects both the factors that make up good nutrition—quality, quantity, and timing—and the obesity epidemic. Logically, we would expect a poor economy to result in a reduction in food consumption and, therefore, a decrease in the number of overweight people. But here in the United States, the increase in the price of high-quality foods may be contributing to increased consumption of low-quality foods. When we add up the cost of buying fresh food, the time it takes to prepare it, and the fact that it tends to spoil quickly, the math favors a visit to the nearest fast-food joint, where a meal is cheap and easy to acquire. Food preparers alter their recipes by adding cheaper ingredients in order to cut costs. For example, soup manufacturers substitute less expensive filler such as carbohydrates for portions of protein such as meat and fish. This cost-savings mentality actually perpetuates the obesity epidemic.

Another important factor contributing to the epidemic is the restaurant industry. Notice how restaurants compete with one another

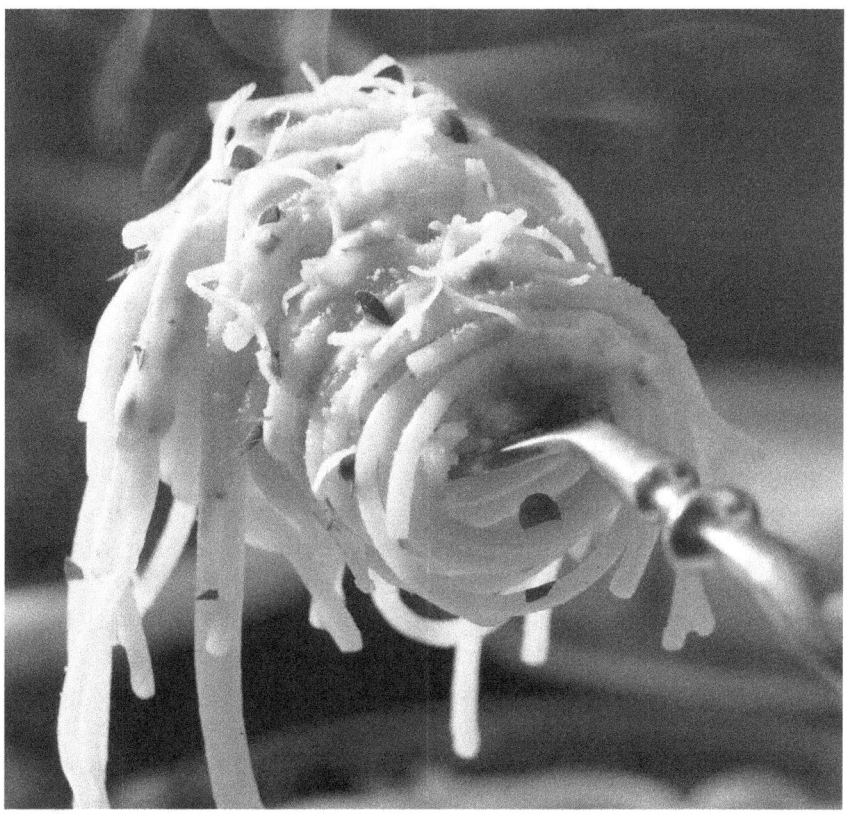

by offering larger portions. An Italian-style restaurant may offer a larger than usual serving of a favorite dish by increasing the amount of pasta and decreasing the amount of protein. If we order spaghetti with meatballs or pasta with seafood, for example, the amount of pasta per serving may be enough to feed an entire family, while the number of shrimp we may be able to count on one hand. If we order an entrée of meat with side dishes, we will find the entrée disproportionately small compared to the size of the plate and the high-carbohydrate sides. In doing this, the restaurant satisfies the customer with large servings while saving money by providing cheaper ingredients. Over time, we become accustomed to seeing more food on our plates, and our stomachs need a larger volume of food to achieve a feeling of satiety. Overeating becomes a way of living; the quality of the food is not a consideration, and before we know it, we have lost our sense of taste and our dignity when it comes to eating habits.

I want to bring in my own Spanish experience for comparison. Spaniards value their food dearly; eating is a ritual and people still schedule their days around meal breaks. Quality is of first importance; they don't just eat anything available. They prefer to eat small portions of good quality food rather than indulge in large portions of junk food. Because meals are scheduled, everyone expects and is expected to gather around the table rather than eat on the go. Spaniards typically follow the three key components for good nutrition, and their rates of obesity and cardiovascular disorders are still low compared to those in the United States. In Spain, the fast-food restaurant industry finds its main clientele among the very young. The core of the population will not replace good food with fast food. The Spanish-language newspaper La Nueva España recently published that the economic crisis is causing a nearly 60 percent decrease in the number of citizens who eat out. There are plenty of restaurants able to prepare quality fish, meats, and legumes, but since good food is becoming more expensive, people cannot afford to visit those restaurants as often. Their alternative is to stay home and cook the food themselves. The fast-food option doesn't seem to be a viable one for the majority of the population.

This is very different from what we do here in the United States. We work hard and we work fast. There is no time for a daily trip to the grocery store, no time for food preparation, and no way we can afford to waste food—or so we think. Instead, we waste our health. Television ads remind us that for five dollars, we can have a whopping meal for two consisting of large amounts of carbohydrates and artery-clogging hydrogenated oils and preservatives, together with an all-you-can-drink soda.

A Lesson from Nature

A couple of years ago, I was giving a talk at a local high school to a group of parents and students. It was an informal setting that allowed the audience to ask questions at any point. I was making a few points about the quality of the food we should eat and comparing what we should do with what the fast-food restaurants offer. At one point I mentioned breastfeeding, and how nature provides us with quality food from the get-go. One of the students raised his hand requesting to ask a question. His comment was this: "Dr. Katalenas, you just made a point in favor of fast food. Breast milk has all the characteristics of fast food; it is fast, cheap, and convenient."

I must confess this adolescent's wit caught me by surprise. But I came up with a response that was seconded by all the parents in the audience, especially the mothers who have breastfed babies. Let's analyze the adjectives one by one:

Breastfeeding is FAST—really? That can be said only by someone who never breastfed. Breastfeeding takes longer than giving babies a bottle, and because breast milk is so easy to digest, the feedings occur more often during the day and night.

CHEAP? Tell that to the millions of mothers in the world who give up working hours and big salaries in order to commit to giving their babies the best nutrition possible because they understand the importance those nutrients have in the development of their baby's body and mind.

AVAILABLE? Not really. Mothers of newborns sacrifice attending events and outings because they know their baby may demand a feeding in the middle of it. Many who don't feel that comfortable breastfeeding in public stay home with our babies on numerous occasions because we understand the importance of giving the best when the best is needed.

Breastfeeding is neither fast, cheap, nor available. And yet every day millions of women make the commitment to breastfeed based purely on the scientifically proven facts that tell them they are making the best choice.

Why then do we stop after breastfeeding? Why is it that parents of toddlers no longer have the quality-quantity-timing mentality that guided them through the first year of the life of their children and throw all that good criteria and common sense out the window the moment the child starts eating table food? Why?

Advertising has a lot to do with the decisions we make in our life. My preference would be for parents to ask their pediatricians and follow their advice before buying the multiple vitamin-added, "good-for-you," packaged food presented to them every time they turn on the television.

A patient of mine, a few years ago, asked me if it was a good idea to offer her four-year-old "fruit snacks" for her mid-afternoon meal. I said, "Yes, sure, fruit is an excellent snack." I then learned what she was referring to when she pulled out of her bag a few pieces of what looked like candy to me.

I now must make this point strongly:

IF IT DOES NOT LOOK LIKE FRUIT—THE WAY IT COMES FROM THE TREE—IT IS NOT A FRUIT.

My desire for families is that they would preserve that breast-feeding mentality, which all parents seem to have at the beginning, throughout their children's entire lives. Rather than allow the advertising industry to tell us how we should feed our children, let's do what's right and let the food industry and the entrepreneurs follow us!

Helpful Tips

— Think about how food looks in nature before offering your family a packaged version of it.
— Plan your meals and work the rest of your schedule around them, making time to prepare and eat without stress.
— Fresh fruit is always a good option for a mid-afternoon snack; it travels well and can be offered anywhere.
— Make the picnic basket part of your travels with the kids.

Chapter 5

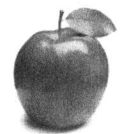 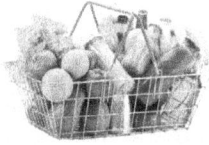 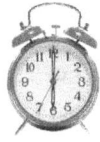

The Fat Lie

The science behind how our bodies react to different nutrients and why we grow and function better when we adopt a healthy lifestyle is beyond the scope of this book, but a few words need to be said about fats, since they have been blamed for the epidemic of obesity. As a result, some have radically eliminated them from their diets, only to load up on empty calories, usually from carbohydrates, while still failing to lose weight.

Next time you visit your favorite grocery store, stroll through the aisle where all the snacks are kept. Count, if you can, the labels indicating "fat-free" or "low-fat" products. I don't want to sound insensitive, but when you look around at your fellow shoppers, tell me whether we as a society have done anything at all to decrease the fat accumulating in our bodies.

One must define terms accurately if we want to truly confront the problem and come up with solutions. We must be mature enough and brave enough to face up to our failure, in spite of all the "fat-free" food we buy, to curb the obesity epidemic.

Facts About Fats

Fat is an important component of our bodies that we cannot afford to ignore. Our brains are made of cholesterol, and our whole nervous system is covered by sheaths of fat. It is integral to the development of children as their skills progress from birth until they reach adult life. The development process includes the formation of millions of neurons and their connections, and also the myelination of nerves, the process by which the nerves acquire a wrapping of fat that allows for more sophisticated functions. Fats carry some liposoluble vitamins such as vitamin D, A, K, and E, which act as antioxidants and are part of cell membranes.

Fat intake should account for about 30 percent of one's diet. However, not all fats behave the same way in our bodies. For health purposes, it is important to understand the differences, so we are going to separate them into two categories, animal fats and vegetable fats. The discrepancies are found in the fatty acid composition; fatty acids are the individual components of a fat and are made up of carbon and hydrogen atoms.

Saturated fats are those present in animal sources such as meats. They have all their carbon atoms saturated by a hydrogen atom; that is, each carbon holds all the hydrogen it can handle without double bonds.

Unsaturated fats have double bonds in between carbon atoms, making the bond tighter and preventing rotation. Unsaturated fats are mostly present in vegetable sources.

Within unsaturated fats, there are cis-unsaturated fats and trans-unsaturated fats. "Cis" and "trans" are terms that refer to the isomer configuration, or chemical-spatial structure, of the molecules. In the cis fatty acid configuration, the hydrogen atoms are located on the same side of the double bond, resulting in a liquid form when at room temperature. Most naturally occurring fatty acids are in the cis configuration.

Trans fatty acids are commercially formed by heating vegetable oil in the presence of metal and hydrogen atoms. Their structure is such that the carbon atoms next to the double bond are on opposite sides, giving them a straighter structure that results in their turning to a solid when at room temperature.

These modified vegetable oils, or trans-unsaturated fats, are used most often in commercial cooking. The process starts out with a vegetable oil that is already chemically processed and altered. It is then hydrogenated: some of the double bonds of the unsaturated oil are broken in order to introduce hydrogen atoms, creating a saturated fat. It is then classified as a trans fat, and is no longer of the cis configuration found in natural vegetable oils.

Why do we bother putting perfectly good vegetable oils through the chemical process of transformation? For convenience and economy: hydrogenated oils containing trans fats are more stable and resist spoilage. Foods manufactured with natural olive oil, for example, could not be stored in our pantries for months. Natural vegetable oils become rancid and change flavor, while hydrogenated oils last much longer. Also, many vegetable oils, olive oil being a good example, burn at fairly low temperatures. Fast-food restaurants use commercial fryers that heat the oil to very high temperatures; hydrogenated oils are capable of withstanding the heat without burning. In summary, the food industry uses hydrogenated oils because they are cheaper and easier to work with.

Recommendations vary regarding fat consumption and the suggested ratio of saturated versus unsaturated fat. We all agree, however, that a healthy diet is one that is low in fat (30 percent of the daily intake of calories, or less), and particularly low in saturated fat and cholesterol. The American Heart Association suggests using unhydrogenated oils and points out how trans fatty acids and hydrogenated oils not only increase bad cholesterol (LDL) but also manage to decrease good cholesterol (HDL), the result of which is an increased risk of cardiovascular disease. Some studies have even found an increased incidence of breast cancer in women with higher levels of trans fatty acids in their adipose tissue.

Case Scenario: Catherine

An eight-year-old girl, Catherine, is sent home from school after an obesity screening with a note from the nurse indicating that she has an elevated body mass index (BMI) that places her above the 95th percentile. We are going to talk about BMI later, but let me say here it is an acceptable and quick way to assess risk for obesity.

Catherine's parents review her current eating habits and make a list of what she is eating regularly. It goes as follows: breakfast consists of two prepackaged toaster pastries and chocolate milk. She eats a midmorning snack of pretzels and juice. Her school lunch typically consists of pizza and juice. She also attends an after-school program where, three days a week, she is given a granola bar and some orange juice, and on the other two days, she is given pre-packaged lunch meat and cheese with juice. When she arrives home at five o'clock in the evening, Catherine likes to snack on potato chips until her seven o'clock dinner time. Her parents prepare a home-cooked meal every night, but Catherine doesn't usually like what is offered, so she eats a small portion and excuses herself from the table to watch TV. Since she never eats a decent dinner, she is always hungry again before bedtime. Her parents offer her some sugary cereal with milk. Sound familiar?

By now, it is obvious what is wrong with this picture: Catherine is eating too much processed food and too little *real* whole food—the kind that contains all-natural ingredients. Although not all packaged food is made the same, to the untrained eye it is really difficult to tell the differences. In general, if an item's list of ingredients is large and it includes some things you can't even pronounce, the advice is to replace the item with a more "natural" one.

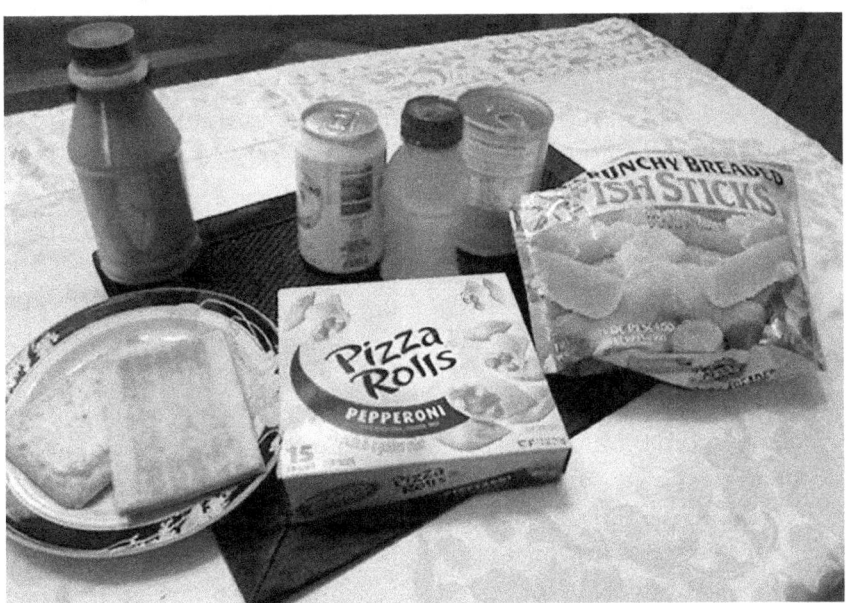

In addition to eating the wrong kinds of food, Catherine is also probably eating too much. Intervention should be geared not only at restructuring her schedule of meals, but also at giving her more real food in smaller amounts and asking her to get some form of exercise, perhaps by playing outside, in the afternoons.

Breakfast could be a slice of toast with real cheese and a few grapes with a glass of milk, for example. Her lunch should include some meat or fish with vegetables, another piece of fruit, and milk to drink. She should be limited to one afternoon snack, and a good choice for a snack would be any kind of fresh fruit or yogurt. Beyond that, there should not be any more food offered until dinnertime, when she should be served a home-cooked meal. Because she will not have been eating continuously throughout the day, she should be hungry and therefore eat her dinner.

Helpful Tips

— Home-prepared foods that are made from scratch are going to contain less chemically altered oils and other ingredients than prepackaged foods.

— A few keywords to look for when checking the ingredients of our food are those of the polyunsaturated fatty acids (PUFA) such as Omega 3 and Omega 6 fatty acids. These are ingredients you want to have in your diet.

— Any food containing the word "hydrogenated" in the list of ingredients has been prepared with chemically altered oils, even if it claims to be "natural."

— Also essential are DHA (docosahexaenoic acid) and ARA (arachidonic acid), fatty acids key to the development of the brain and eyes. For that reason, they are now a component of infant formulas.

— The beneficial effects of fish oil, which is rich in PUFAs, extend beyond the first year of life. Studies show a valuable outcome when older children are given supplements of fish oil, the primary benefit being an improvement of the immune system that results in a decreased occurrence of bronchitis, bronchiolitis, and febrile illnesses.

Part II

The Solution

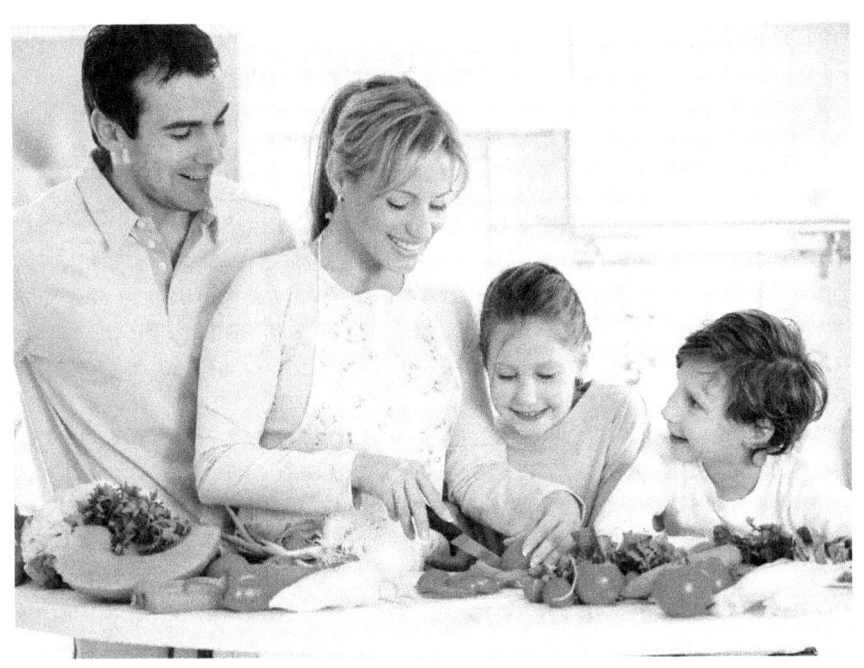

On July 17, 1996, Trans World Airlines (TWA) Flight 800 from New York to Paris exploded and crashed into the Atlantic Ocean killing all 230 people on board. I remember the day vividly. I was living in New Jersey at the time with my husband and our small children. I very much related to all those families going through the agony of having no answers to so many questions: What happened? Who did it? Was it an accident?

A couple of years later, when I flew into New York's LaGuardia Airport, my plane landed some distance from our gate and had to cruise through long strips of tarmac in order to get to the terminal. From my small window view, I caught a glimpse of several hangar buildings on our way to the gate. I happened to open a magazine in front of me and a picture caught my eye. It was a picture of a hangar door wide-open, just like the ones I could see from my window, and inside was what resembled an airplane, pieces missing, glued together in an attempt to reconstruct the original shape. As I read the story, I found out it was TWA Flight 800; they had fished pieces of the plane out of the ocean off the coast of Long Island, one by one, and they had reconstructed the aircraft almost entirely, in an attempt to find the cause of the accident. As I kept looking out at the hangars nearby, I imagined the airplane inside one of them, with hundreds of people working to reconstruct it piece after piece, and I imagined how much effort that entailed, searching for an answer. I still get a knot in my throat when I recall this memory.

What amazes me the most about the American way is the tenacity, the capacity to organize endeavors in order to reach a goal, and the fact that no effort is spared despite adversity. It doesn't matter the cost; if it is worthwhile, we Americans get it done.

Knowing what we have been capable of throughout history, I am convinced that we can analyze and confront the obesity epidemic once we put our minds to it—even if it involves changing our lifestyles and habits. I know that once we understand the importance and the need to eat less and better, we are going to join efforts and successfully increase the life expectancy of our children and grandchildren. Gradually, the restaurant industry, which is part of the capitalist system that answers to consumer demand, is going to cater to our needs and give us the healthy food choices we are asking for. But first, we must be able to identify what in our daily lives is good and healthy and what is not; we must be able to familiarize our families with how to tell the difference. Lasting changes typically requires long efforts.

Chapter 6

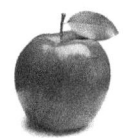 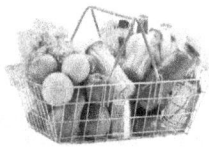 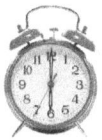

Exercise

No book dedicated to giving healthy advice would be complete without mentioning exercise. Here's my quick and to-the-point summary of the exercise dilemma: we are not doing enough, and we all know it. But how can that be our reality in a country with such excellent sports and recreation facilities? Our schools spend millions of dollars providing exercise equipment, sports fields built to code; neighborhoods take pride in building walking and bike trails; and parents try very hard to get kids into elite teams, often spending large sums of money in the effort. So, it is not lack of knowledge about the benefits of an active lifestyle; it is not lack of access to exercise. What is it? Where are we doing wrong?

I am going to illustrate different real-life situations to explain the problem and formulate the solution:

Case Scenario: Justin

Justin is a nine-year-old boy with a BMI over the 95th percentile. He lives with his parents and two younger siblings, a two-year-old sister and a seven-year-old brother. Mom and dad work outside of the home. Every day after school he goes to an after-school day care where he plays indoors with other kids until 5:30 .m., when his mother picks him and his brother up, after stopping at the daycare his sister attends. When they arrive home, his mother engages in food preparation while Justin and his brother do their homework. He has no friends around the neighborhood, since most of the kids are younger than he is. His parents don't feel comfortable allowing him to play outside by himself because of safety concerns. After dinner he plays video games and watches TV before going to bed. He must get to bed early, since he has to get up early enough for parents to take his sister to day care before school starts. On Saturdays they usually visit grandparents outside of town and go shopping in the car or run errands around town. By Sunday, the parents are tired and spend the day doing laundry, resting, and getting ready for the week.

When it comes to identifying the main problem keeping us from exercising, this family is typical. We just don't have the opportunity to exercise as part of our normal daily activities. Our errands require use of a car and involve trips to different parts of town, too far to walk. They may be doing everything right as far as eating

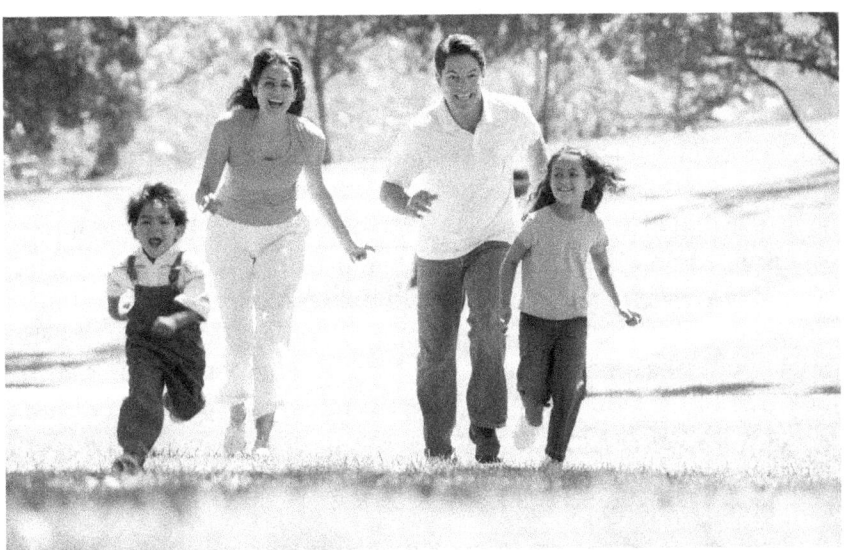

habits are concerned, cooking meals at home and keeping to a meal schedule.

The solution for this family involved finding a one-hour period each day when they could engage in an exercise activity. Mother started following the one-week menu described in this book, and by doing that she was able to limit the time spent cooking, since she started preparing some of the meals on Sunday evening. She then started taking the three kids to a park near their house at 5:30 p.m.; she parked the car and allowed them to play for an hour. Then they all walked home (about one mile), leaving the car at the park. By the time they got home, Justin's dad was starting dinner, which both parents finished together while the older children did their homework.

After dinner they all walked to the park to pick up the car, this time bringing the dog along. They got home in time for bath and bed. At bedtime the children were tired and able to fall asleep fast, allowing the parents some time to relax alone. They also scheduled some outside activity for Saturday, involving the grandparents in the outing. On Sunday, one parent did the errands while the other spent time at the park with the children.

The message here is that you don't need to be athletically oriented or pay money to remain physically active. But it does take a desire to change and a commitment to change, in order to do so without adding more work to an already busy life.

Case Scenario: Megan and Kyle

Megan and Kyle are a sister and brother ten and thirteen years old, respectively. They attend elementary and middle school and are doing well academically. Each has a BMI over the 85th percentile.

Their dad is a coach of Kyle's baseball and football elite teams, and their mother teaches Megan tennis, her favorite sport. They practice every day of the week, and they have tournaments during the weekends. The mom does not work outside of the home, but gives tennis lessons to children and adults two days a week. Since they live in the country, they have to drive long distances in and out of town to go to school and attend practice. Tournaments are usually out of town, which requires them to spend weekends gone from home for long periods.

They don't have time to cook meals at home. They usually buy fast food and often eat in the car in between activities.

For this family, lack of exercise is not the problem. If anything, they were exercising a lot, without taking time out to relax, engage in free play, or really enjoy their time together. They was also spending a lot of extra money to participate on the various teams and were all constantly tired.

The solution for this family came when they balanced their life and realized they were putting out so much effort to remain active but yet still were receiving a diagnosis of obesity. It was hard for the parents to admit the problem; they didn't think they "deserved" it, since exercising was of such importance to them. It is important to mention that both parents were found to have an increased Body Mass Index, when they checked with their own doctor.

The change they introduced involved quitting their elite teams and playing for fun only. The kids started having friends over to play in their large backyard, and soon they were having more fun with less effort. Mom now had time to dedicate to shopping for food and cooking a meal every day. She made a meal schedule for the week and kept a watch on portion size. She eliminated sports drinks and offered the kids water when they were thirsty.

Since the parents enjoyed the outdoors, they had no trouble finding places to take their children on weekends; they found a variety of different activities, from rock climbing and swimming to paintball, hiking, and dancing. One year after the lifestyle change, each of the children was able to identify his or her own favorite activity, rather than just following what the parents made them do. Soon Megan indicated her preference for dance lessons, and she signed up for once a week classes. Kyle kept trying different activities every week, without committing to any in particular. They continued to remain active while at the same time finding more enjoyment in the activities and also improving their eating habits.

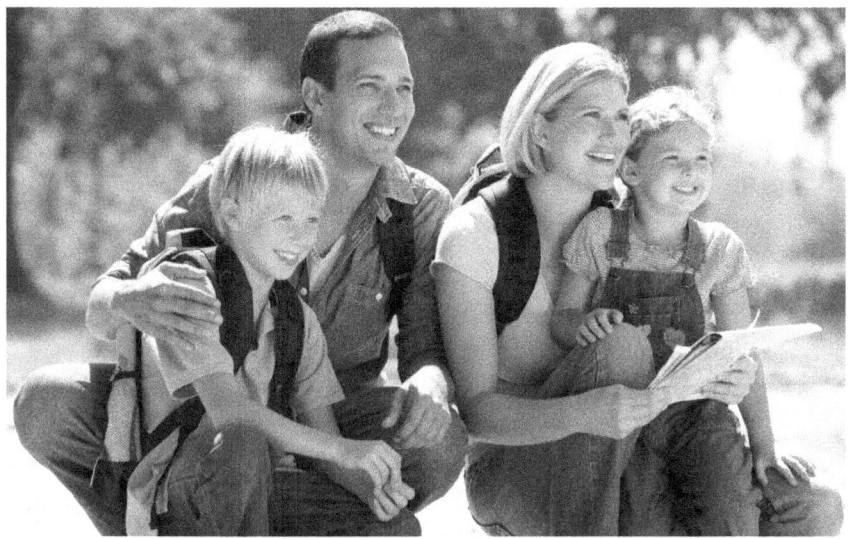

Case Scenario: David

David is a twelve-year-old who does not enjoy outdoor activities. He is into technology and gaming; he can spend hours in front of the computer or console. He takes part in one hour of PE every day at school, but he spends most of his free time playing video games. His parents are so busy working that they don't have much time to dedicate to outside activities. David lives in a neighborhood of kids who often come to his door to ask him to play, but he prefers to stay in the house. Because his BMI has climbed above the 85th percentile, his parents knew they needed to find a way to increase his activity level.

The solution came with two very simple rules adopted by the family. David's school is about three-fourths of a mile from their house; the parents started getting him out of bed a little earlier in the morning and walking with him to school. His mother still picked him up after school because she was afraid to allow him to walk home alone. After a couple of weeks of walking to school, he met other children from the neighborhood who attended the same school and who also walked to school. He actually started to enjoy the morning walk. Soon he asked his mother not to pick him up after school, since he preferred to walk home with his new friends.

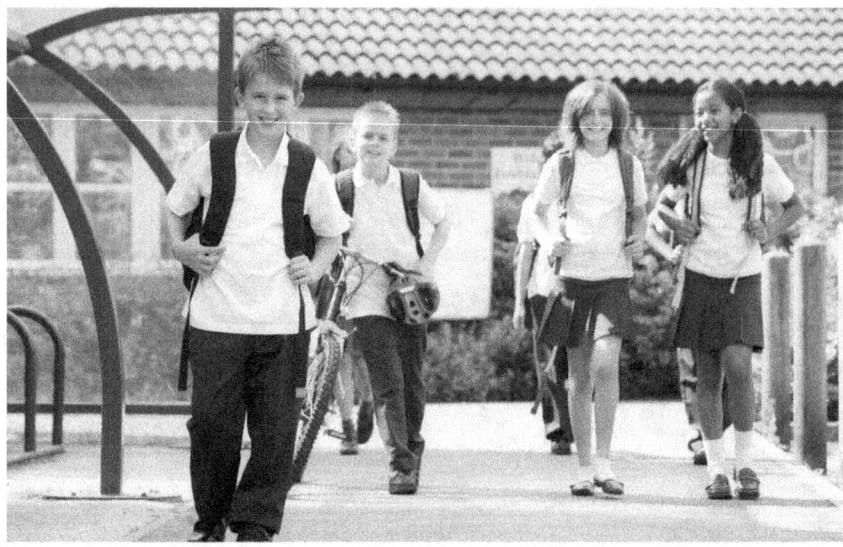

The parents also started limiting David's "screen time" to one hour a day on school nights and two hours on weekends. Forced to find something else to do with his time, he started going out and seeking the company of other children to engage in free play. His parents now have a different problem: he spends too much time outside and doesn't want to come home in the evenings.

Let's Get Physical

In most places in the United States, many of our daily tasks and errands require a car and consume a lot of time. We have to be creative in order to spend more of our time engaged in physical movement.

On top of that, physical education is not required in some schools and for certain grades, and even when it is required, some children don't even exercise the way they should during PE. Some students tell me they just walk around the field and don't even break a sweat.

I remember watching my own middle boy, when he was in elementary school, walking behind a group of running kids during a "running club" activity. He was engaged in what appeared to be a deep discussion with another kid. When I asked him what was so important to discuss when they were supposed to be running, he informed me they were talking about the stock market! While the incident was funny and we still remember it at family gatherings, the truth is that too many kids can get by without expending much energy during PE. Therefore, they come home from school still in need of an environment conducive to staying active.

Parents must realize that a small change is better than no change at all and come up with creative solutions to their children's need for exercise. The good news is that children respond much better than adults to such lifestyle changes; you'll be surprised by the results once you set some new rules and stick to them.

Helpful Tips

— Take the children to the park every day and allow free play. It provides a great opportunity to make friends with other parents or to get some reading done, if your kids are old enough that you don't have to observe them continuously.
— Find a neighborhood newspaper that lists activities available on the weekends.
— Park you car and walk home. Go back and pick up the car after dinner.
— Walk your dog around the block; make your children responsible for exercising the dog if they are old enough to do it themselves.
— Walk your kids to school.
— Encourage activities after school, trying different ones until you discover what your children enjoy.
— Limit screen time to one hour a day. Children will have to find something else to do, and they will use their imagination in the process.
— If you live in a safe neighborhood, allow your kids to play outside with friends. Invite their friends to visit your children and ask them to play outside.
— Older kids may enjoy gardening, mowing the lawn, or washing your car.
— Many neighborhoods have recreation centers with activities for all ages. Find out what is available and make use of community resources.

Chapter 7

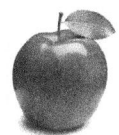 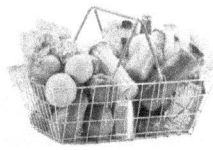 

Why Some People Are Skinny and Some Are Not

The Thrifty Genotype Theory

We all have relatives and friends who don't seem to gain weight under any circumstances. They can eat what they want without suffering any consequences—at least, any that are visible—while others of us seem to feel the fat deposit as we swallow.

The explanation is simple: genes. Our genetic makeup determines how our bodies handle the energy we consume in the form of food. The body needs energy intake on a regular basis in order to maintain the function of the organs. The brain, for example, needs constant access to glucose, which explains why we feel light-headed and can faint if our blood sugar falls below a certain level. The energy also ensures that our livers continue to function, it enables the digestive system to produce the substances that aid digestion, and it makes our muscles and bones supportive and mobile. At a minimum, we have a metabolic need for food in order to maintain a normal weight. Heavier people have a higher metabolic need because it takes more energy to move a body mass of 300 pounds than it does to move a body weighing only 150 pounds.

Well, this part is easy to understand. But what happens when we consume more than we need to maintain the basics? Our bodies are genetically programmed to be "thrifty"—to store excess energy in the form of adipose tissue and lean muscle. That is, we accumulate fat and protein, the proportions of which are determined by our genes. Historically, those who were prone to the accumulation of fat had the advantage of being resistant to the negative effects of starvation and, therefore, were better able to survive during periods of undernourishment. Some ethnic groups, for example, such as the Pima Indians in the United States, have an increased commonness of this "thrifty" genetic makeup that, for generations, has allowed them to survive periods of starvation and food scarcity. Today, due to an increase in sedentary lifestyle and food intake, they have one of the highest incidences of obesity and diabetes. In other words, because of their genetic predisposition, they should be eating less and exercising more in order to offset their natural tendency to accumulate fat. The phenomenon of the "thrifty genotype" is an interesting one. It means that those of us who possess genes capable of saving energy in the form of fat need to pay closer attention to what and when we eat, and to engage in daily physical exercise in order to maintain balance.

Another interesting concept is the nutrient environment in utero and its impact on weight gain later in life. Certain studies conducted during World War II showed that pregnant women who were suffering from severe undernutrition gave birth to children who were more likely to be obese as adults. The causality is poorly understood, but it seems to be that the scarcity of nutrients in utero manages to program the energy-processing capability, so that those infants tend to accumulate energy in the form of fat, almost as if the body were anticipating future shortages.

Something similar happens to premature babies, who have an increased incidence of obesity later in life. The explanation is the same: the body, deprived of time to assimilate nutrients from the mother, sets in place a mechanism of energy accumulation that lasts a lifetime. People who were born prematurely, therefore, must be very careful to establish good eating and exercise habits from early on in order to counterbalance their natural tendency to accumulate fat.

To top it off, we recognize that genes are also responsible for impulse control. We all know families in which alcoholism, for example, is found among members of several generations. Just as alcoholism is a result, in part, of being genetically predisposed to poor impulse control, so is overeating.

However, we can't blame it all on genetics. The environment is influential as well. Even people with a "thrifty genotype" and poor impulse control, if placed in a healthy environment where consistent portions of nutritious food are available on a set schedule, can be successful in controlling their weight.

Creating a Healthy Food Environment:

— Establish healthy eating habits early in life
— Prepare small portions of food
— Eliminate snacking
— Create a schedule of meals and eat only at mealtime
— Perform physical exercise for at least one hour every day
— Limit television and computer time to no more than two hours per day

What Happens If We Don't Improve Our Eating Habits?

Data indicate that we are not moving in the right direction. In the United States, the consumption of snacks and fast food has increased over the last twenty years. We have also seen an increase in portion size and a decrease in physical exercise. This, combined with a prevalence of individuals with a "thrifty genotype," is responsible for the present situation: the emergence of chronic illnesses in youth due to obesity.

Cardiovascular disease, diabetes, and the conditions that precede them are among those illnesses. Elevated blood pressure and high cholesterol, for example, are more common in adolescents who are obese; the presence of elevated lipids and blood pressure during childhood increases the risk of cardiovascular disease during adulthood. The initial process involved in atherosclerosis, or hardening of the arteries, begins in childhood with the formation of fibrous plaque, a deposition of fat tissue inside the arteries. When the plaque eventually causes obstruction of blood flow, it either affects the blood vessels of the heart, making one vulnerable to heart attack, or it affects the blood vessels of the brain, making one vulnerable to stroke.

A New Disease Is Emerging: Metabolic Syndrome

During the last decade, a completely new syndrome has been added to the list of diseases affecting the young: metabolic syndrome, or syndrome X. It is so new that the medical community lacks consensus regarding the components of the condition. In essence, though, metabolic syndrome is a combination of signs and symptoms that together leads to cardiovascular disease and diabetes. It is diagnosed when an individual presents at least three of the five following symptoms:

— Waist circumference is larger than 102 centimeters in men and larger than 88 centimeters in women.

— Triglycerides are higher than 150 milligrams per deciliter.
— HDL (good cholesterol) is lower than 40 milligrams per deciliter in men and lower than 50 milligrams per deciliter in women.
— Blood pressure is higher than 130 over 85.
— Fasting glucose level (blood sugar level before a meal) is higher than 100 milligrams per deciliter.

Another, more obvious sign of trouble that has prompted schools to screen children in recent years is a change in the coloration and texture of the skin, most visible around the neck, underarms, and lower abdomen. It is known as acanthosis nigricans (AN) and is a sign of insulin resistance and an indication of predisposition to diabetes.

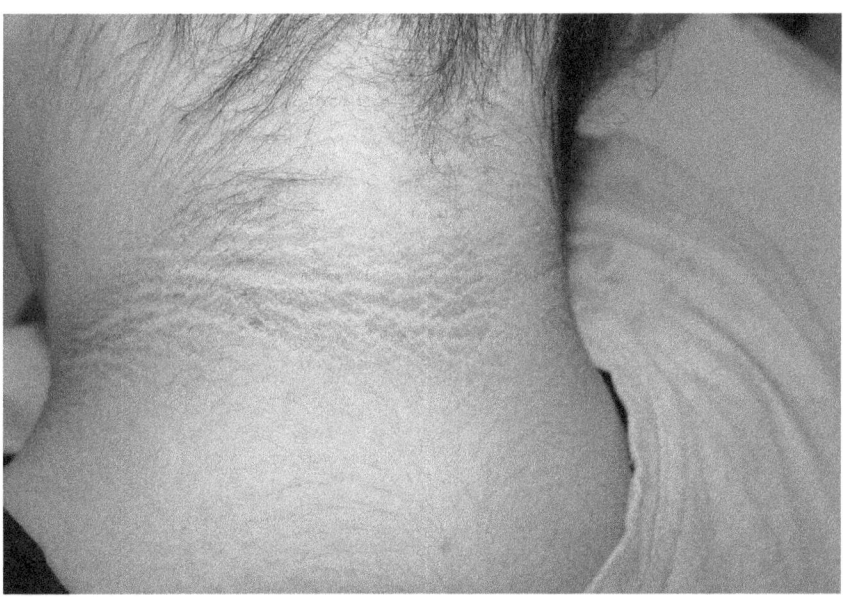

School nurses are well trained to identify students with AN, and they instruct families to check with their pediatricians to determine what steps to follow. When a child is identified as having AN, a series of laboratory studies should be performed to determine the level of cholesterol and other lipids, to check blood pressure, and to calculate the child's body mass index (BMI). If and when AN is determined to be associated with obesity, the child should undergo intervention to start a weight-management program.

Chapter 8

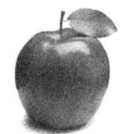 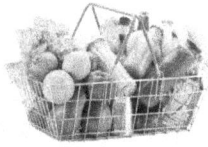 

Body Mass Index

Perception, Perception, Perception

When I was a little girl, I used to watch *Bonanza*, the TV show, every week. It used to air on Sunday afternoon in Spain, during the 1960s. No matter what the plan was for the day, I had to make time for my favorite show. (Remember, we didn't have VCRs, DVRs, or television on-demand back then.) It was loyalty, pure and simple, that you had to demonstrate when you liked a TV program.

Kids my age, both boys and girls, enjoyed the show. Boys were thrilled with the Wild West environment of the stories, and the girls loved "Little Joe," played by Michael Landon. My take was a bit different; I really liked Hoss Cartwright, played by Dan Blocker. He portrayed the middle son of the Cartwright family; a not-so-bright, huge guy who was the target of innocent jokes by his brothers. It was the consensus back then that Hoss was a big person, bigger than the average citizen and, therefore, was noticeable for that reason alone. I was touched by his gentle style, and to me, he represented the good, the sweet, the innocent . . . OK, I had a Hoss crush.

Nowadays, I watch *Bonanza* on TV Land when I have the opportunity. I remember some of the episodes from forty years ago, but I observe the stories and the characters through different eyes. Hoss, my favorite character, is not fat anymore. I now see him as a tall person of average weight, when a few decades ago this character was practically obese, no doubt about it.

I then did a little experiment at home. I asked my three children what they thought of Hoss, after watching a few minutes of the show. I wanted to know if they considered the character to be thin, average, or obese. I was surprised to learn that all three of my kids consider a person weighing three hundred pounds "average." That was their unanimous opinion, which matches my own.

My point is that today we are accustomed to seeing overweight people everywhere. This changes the perception of "normal," and it makes it more difficult to recognize the problem in ourselves and in our kids. If we don't even see the issue, how are we going to fix it?

Here is a way to tell if you or your child is overweight when compared to other children his or her age. It is called the Body Mass Index and is usually measured by pediatricians at the time of wellness exams after five years of age. It is easy to calculate, and you can do it at home without difficulty just following a few directions.

The BMI Calculation

Body mass index (BMI), a calculation that uses height and weight to estimate how much body fat someone has, is a simple tool used to determine the risk for obesity in both adults and children. BMI is calculated by dividing weight in pounds by height in inches squared, and then multiplying by 703. For example, if a ten-year-old girl weighs 66 pounds and is 55 inches tall, in order to calculate her BMI, we first find the square of her height which is 3,025 (55 X 55). Next, we divide 66 by 3,025, which equals .0218. We then simply multiply this last number by 703; the result is a BMI of 15.3. Once determined, we can see how the BMI correlates with either "normal" readings or "overweight/obese" readings.

Because for children BMI changes as they grow, a BMI percentile is used for purposes of comparison to other children of the same age and gender. To compare a child's BMI to that of other children, we consult a table like the ones found here (see figs. 8.1 and 8.2). The pink table corresponds to girls' readings, and the blue table to boys' readings.

Now we go to the pink curve and correlate the child's BMI, which is 15.3, with the child's age, which is ten years, and we can see how the BMI falls right below the 50th percentile mark. That is a *normal* value—meaning that the child is not overweight. For children, any value of BMI above the 85th percentile is considered at risk for obesity, and values above the 95th percentile are considered obese. If a child falls into either of these categories, a doctor should be consulted prior to introducing any changes in diet since other diagnostic tests may be required.

Having this information helps in understanding the need for lifestyle changes that will impact a child's overall health. The good news is that moderate weight loss has a significant impact in reducing the odds of developing cardiovascular disease or diabetes. In adults, a modest loss of 5 to 7 percent is successful in preventing diabetes. In children, just maintaining weight during growth in height has a beneficial effect in preventing the development of diabetes. However, consult a physician before starting a child on a weight-loss diet. The key, again, is early intervention and the establishment of good family eating habits from the beginning.

In adults, body mass index is calculated by using the same formula. However, since the BMI in adults does not change with

Figure 8.1

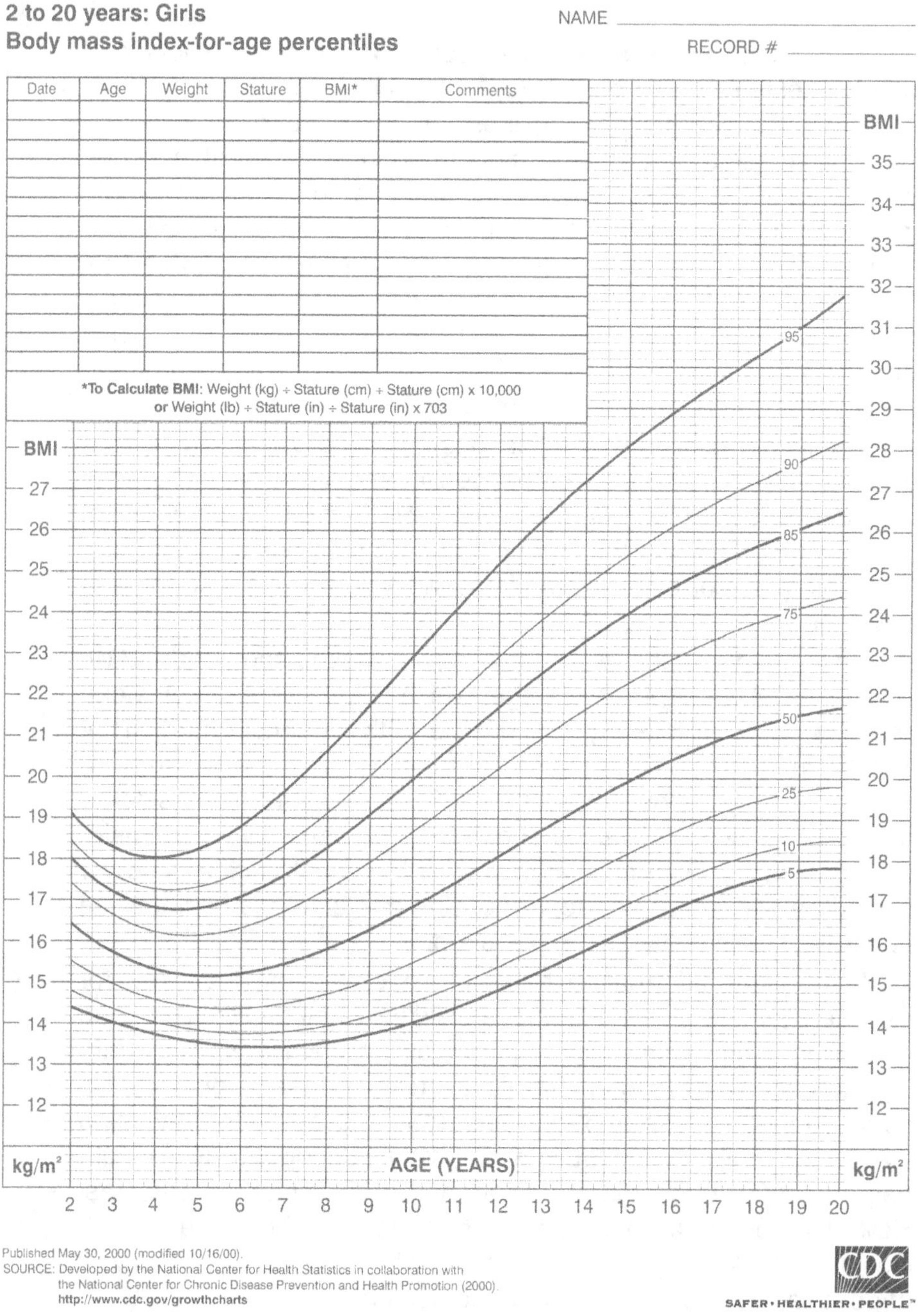
2 to 20 years: Girls
Body mass index-for-age percentiles
NAME
RECORD #
Date
Age
Weight
Stature
BMI*
Comments
*To Calculate BMI: Weight (kg) ÷ Stature (cm) ÷ Stature (cm) x 10,000
or Weight (lb) ÷ Stature (in) ÷ Stature (in) x 703
BMI
95
90
85
75
50
25
10
5
kg/m²
AGE (YEARS)
Published May 30, 2000 (modified 10/16/00).
SOURCE: Developed by the National Center for Health Statistics in collaboration with
the National Center for Chronic Disease Prevention and Health Promotion (2000).
http://www.cdc.gov/growthcharts
CDC
SAFER • HEALTHIER • PEOPLE™

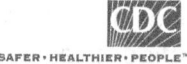

Figure 8.2

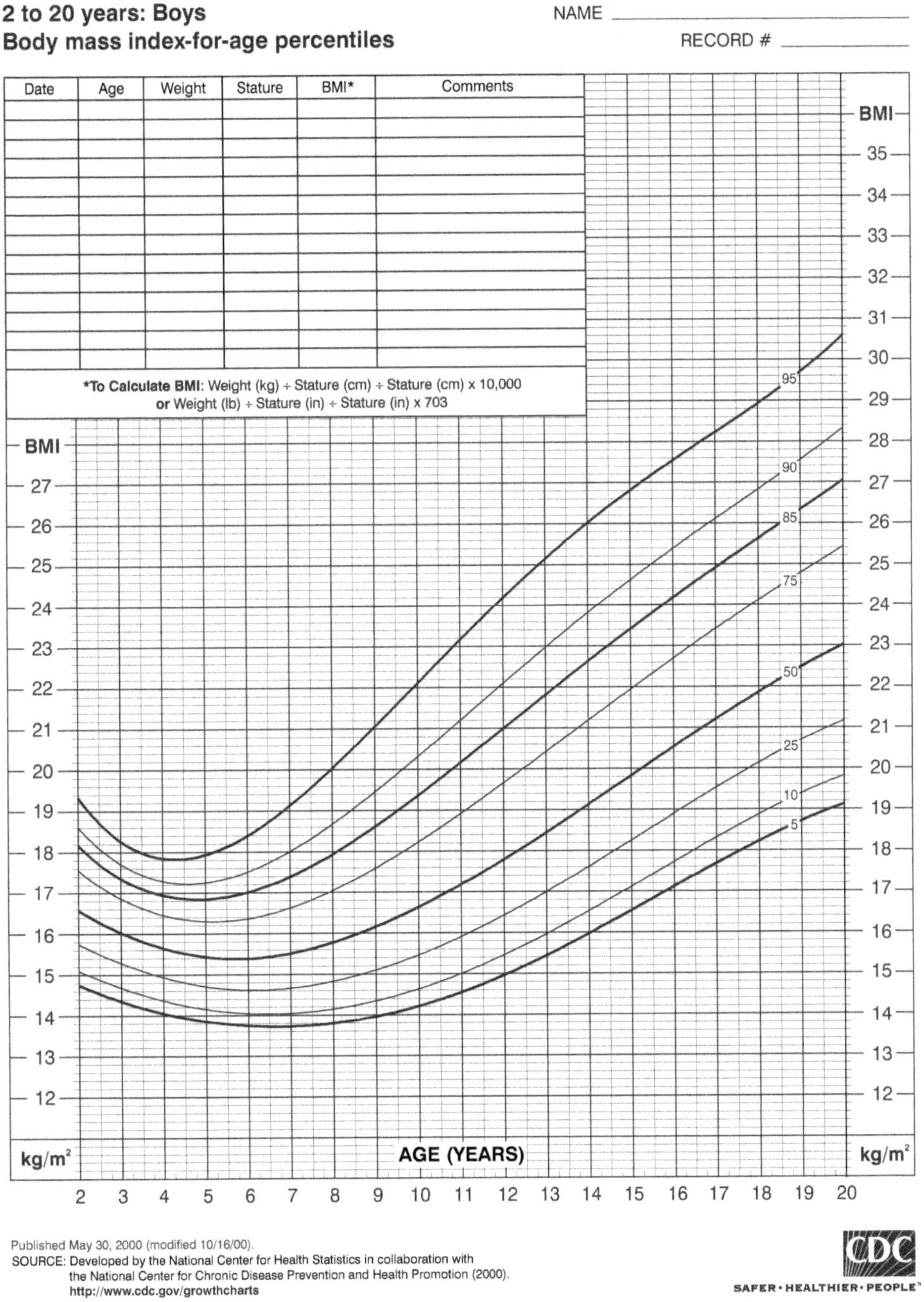

2 to 20 years: Boys
Body mass index-for-age percentiles

NAME _____

RECORD # _____

Date	Age	Weight	Stature	BMI*	Comments

*To Calculate BMI: Weight (kg) ÷ Stature (cm) ÷ Stature (cm) x 10,000
or Weight (lb) ÷ Stature (in) ÷ Stature (in) x 703

BMI

95
90
85
75
50
25
10
5

AGE (YEARS)

kg/m² ... kg/m²

2 3 4 5 6 7 8 9 10 11 12 13 14 15 16 17 18 19 20

Published May 30, 2000 (modified 10/16/00).
SOURCE: Developed by the National Center for Health Statistics in collaboration with
the National Center for Chronic Disease Prevention and Health Promotion (2000).
http://www.cdc.gov/growthcharts

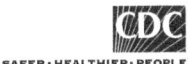

SAFER·HEALTHIER·PEOPLE™

age (because they are full-grown), the number obtained doesn't need to be plotted on a curve as it does in the case of children. The same table is used for males and females. If the number obtained is over 35, the person is considered obese. If the number is between 25 and 35, he or she is at risk for obesity. The ideal BMI for an adult, therefore, is below 25. Table 8.1, Adult Body Mass Index, on the next page, displays the standard data for adults' BMI.

"Mi" Struggle Is "Su" Struggle

Recently, I was talking to a dear friend of mine about her sister who, after having a bilateral knee-replacement surgery months before, continued to suffer in constant pain, requiring pain medication daily. I must explain, it is difficult for a person who is a doctor to separate roles at certain times; as I talk to friends or family members about medical issues, they all expect me to give an opinion that is going to, right away, be elevated to a higher standard than if it came from a layperson. I try my best to direct all such medical questions arising from my direct family and friends to their own doctors, after reminding them they should follow the advice of the physician who knows them well, medically speaking, and possesses the necessary information to give medical advice. But this time I was guided by the distress expressed by my friend, who seemed to be at the end of her rope, after consulting different doctors. It was the general consensus that the surgery had gone well and that the patient should be on her way to recovery by now, without the pain and suffering she was enduring.

After stepping back from the situation, and without knowing the whole story, I ventured to suggest that maybe the delay in recovery was due to the patient's overweight condition. My comment was offered out of an innocent and genuine desire to shed some light on the problem. But it was not taken well. My friend proceeded to tell me that her sister was not overweight, that no doctor ever mentioned she was, and that, therefore, the cause of the pain in her knees could in no way be related to weight. I could feel our friendship shaken by the tone of her voice and the expressions she used to communicate her disapproval of my opinion.

Since I had already started it, I definitely considered finishing my point by explaining it to the end. I pulled out my Body Mass Index chart, and we looked up my friend's sister's numbers. I thus

Table 8.1

Body Mass Index Table

BMI (Height in inches)	Normal						Overweight					Obese										Extreme Obesity															
BMI	19	20	21	22	23	24	25	26	27	28	29	30	31	32	33	34	35	36	37	38	39	40	41	42	43	44	45	46	47	48	49	50	51	52	53	54
																					Body Weight (pounds)															
58	91	96	100	105	110	115	119	124	129	134	138	143	148	153	158	162	167	172	177	181	186	191	196	201	205	210	215	220	224	229	234	239	244	248	253	258
59	94	99	104	109	114	119	124	128	133	138	143	148	153	158	163	168	173	178	183	188	193	198	203	208	212	217	222	227	232	237	242	247	252	257	262	267
60	97	102	107	112	118	123	128	133	138	143	148	153	158	163	168	174	179	184	189	194	199	204	209	215	220	225	230	235	240	245	250	255	261	266	271	276
61	100	106	111	116	122	127	132	137	143	148	153	158	164	169	174	180	185	190	195	201	206	211	217	222	227	232	238	243	248	254	259	264	269	275	280	285
62	104	109	115	120	126	131	136	142	147	153	158	164	169	175	180	186	191	196	202	207	213	218	224	229	235	240	246	251	256	262	267	273	278	284	289	295
63	107	113	118	124	130	135	141	146	152	158	163	169	175	180	186	191	197	203	208	214	220	225	231	237	242	248	254	259	265	270	278	282	287	293	299	304
64	110	116	122	128	134	140	145	151	157	163	169	174	180	186	192	197	204	209	215	221	227	232	238	244	250	256	262	267	273	279	285	291	296	302	308	314
65	114	120	126	132	138	144	150	156	162	168	174	180	186	192	198	204	210	216	222	228	234	240	246	252	258	264	270	276	282	288	294	300	306	312	318	324
66	118	124	130	136	142	148	155	161	167	173	179	186	192	198	204	210	216	223	229	235	241	247	253	260	266	272	278	284	291	297	303	309	315	322	328	334
67	121	127	134	140	146	153	159	166	172	178	185	191	198	204	211	217	223	230	236	242	249	255	261	268	274	280	287	293	299	306	312	319	325	331	338	344
68	125	131	138	144	151	158	164	171	177	184	190	197	203	210	216	223	230	236	243	249	256	262	269	276	282	289	295	302	308	315	322	328	335	341	348	354
69	128	135	142	149	155	162	169	176	182	189	196	203	209	216	223	230	236	243	250	257	263	270	277	284	291	297	304	311	318	324	331	338	345	351	358	365
70	132	139	146	153	160	167	174	181	188	195	202	209	216	222	229	236	243	250	257	264	271	278	285	292	299	306	313	320	327	334	341	348	355	362	369	376
71	136	143	150	157	165	172	179	186	193	200	208	215	222	229	236	243	250	257	265	272	279	286	293	301	308	315	322	329	338	343	351	358	365	372	379	386
72	140	147	154	162	169	177	184	191	199	206	213	221	228	235	242	250	258	265	272	279	287	294	302	309	316	324	331	338	346	353	361	368	375	383	390	397
73	144	151	159	166	174	182	189	197	204	212	219	227	235	242	250	257	265	272	280	288	295	302	310	318	325	333	340	348	355	363	371	378	386	393	401	408
74	148	155	163	171	179	186	194	202	210	218	225	233	241	249	256	264	272	280	287	295	303	311	319	326	334	342	350	358	365	373	381	389	396	404	412	420
75	152	160	168	176	184	192	200	208	216	224	232	240	248	256	264	272	279	287	295	303	311	319	327	335	343	351	359	367	375	383	391	399	407	415	423	431
76	156	164	172	180	189	197	205	213	221	230	238	246	254	263	271	279	287	295	304	312	320	328	336	344	353	361	369	377	385	394	402	410	418	426	435	443

Source: Adapted from Clinical Guidelines on the Identification, Evaluation, and Treatment of Overweight and Obesity in Adults: The Evidence Report.

proved to her that she was indeed above the 95th percentile, which made the stress to her knees more than it should be and, therefore, could contribute to her pain. The story did not end there, as you can imagine. My friend went on to remind me that I always blame everything on obesity, that her whole family is obese, and that there is nothing they can do about it, adding that I only mention it because I am not obese and so don't know what a struggle it is.

I then pulled out the Body Mass Index chart again, and we now looked up *my* numbers, which showed that I need to lose six pounds in order to be where I should be.

It is human nature to avoid painful truths when we are not ready to face our reality. It is also human nature for friends and family to refrain from mentioning the real problem when we know it can cause distress to another person. In an effort to avoid confrontation, we often say what the other person wants to hear, and so it goes. As a result, we now have a society that overlooks and dismisses the obvious because it is too painful to face up to it. The objective eye of your doctor can give you an unbiased opinion when you ask for one; don't dismiss it without giving it consideration. If your friend is a doctor, ask questions at your own risk of receiving the appropriate answer.

A word of advice to my fellow doctors: when you see a patient who is obese, please share your thoughts with him or her, as probably no one else will. Even when weight management is not your specialty, even when the patient may be in front of you for an entirely different reason, use all your compassion to direct the patient to another practitioner who may be able to help, but don't let the opportunity go by without offering your medical opinion. It is too important to let it go unmentioned.

When I see patients in my office, I am not supposed to share my personal experiences and struggles with them. I am there to give professional advice based on evidence and research, devoid of all personal bias. But this is my book, and I feel free to share something with you that I thought should be obvious: we all have struggles, we all have good and bad days, and nobody is perfect. It is called being human. This thought should not keep us from trying every day; it should not keep us from acknowledging what we need to do, learning how to do it, and giving it a shot. That, too, is being human.

I was born with Scheuermann's disease. It is a condition whereby the spine has certain curvatures that are more exaggerated than they should be.For that reason, pain is a given. If my weight goes up just by a couple of pounds, I can feel it in by back. The pain increases and movement becomes more difficult. If I were to then decrease my exercise activity, I would enter into a cycle of pain and weight gain. I try to avoid this at all costs. How? By keeping a constant vigilance and trying to apply the quality-quantity-timing test to my decisions when it comes to food. If I see the pounds accumulating, I return to the starting point. I, too, live in this dietarily dysfunctional culture and am just as exposed to its pernicious influences as anyone else. Being so close to the problem makes me all the more determined to explain the solution that I know works.

Chapter 9

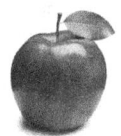 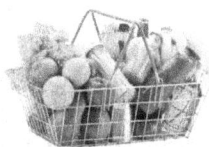 

The Olive Oil Answer

Ever since the discovery of fire, mankind has preferred cooked food. Not long after, we realized that spices, condiments, and oils add to the flavor of a meal. Oil acts as a catalyst to promote consistent cooking, enhance natural flavors, break down sugars, and improve the whole eating experience. But wait … oils are fats! And ours is a society catering to the fat-free culture promoted for decades by a well-intentioned but ill-informed food industry. Yes, oils add to the fat content of the diet; and yes, fats have more calories than other nutrients. But not all oils are made the same, and this brings us back to the relationship between quantity, quality, and timing.

As mentioned previously, oil (fat) produces about 9 calories per gram consumed, compared with the 3 calories per gram produced by carbohydrates, and the 4 calories per gram produced by protein. What this means is that we must consume smaller amounts of fat since it translates into more cumulative calories if not burned through exercise. It doesn't mean, however, that we must eliminate fats altogether. In fact, except for those of us with specific health concerns, 30 percent of our diets should be composed of fat. Let us also remember that in children, their developing nervous systems appreciate the fat content of their diets. After all, the brain is made of cholesterol!

As mentioned in previous chapters, there is good cholesterol and there is bad cholesterol. When we consume too many fats of animal origin, bad cholesterol increases. It then manages to accumulate inside the arteries and contributes to difficulties in the circulation of blood through the blood vessels. If those blood vessels, now obstructed by plaque, happen to be the ones delivering blood to vital organs such as the brain or the heart, we could end up with a serious disorder such as a heart attack or stroke. For this reason, it is of vital importance to make sure that the fat we consume is the kind that will promote the good cholesterol rather than the bad.

The history of olive oil goes back centuries. The olive tree grows well in a variety of temperate climates, such as we find in Mediterranean countries. Ancient cultures attributed superb properties to the oil of the olive, believing it was a source of health, strength, and beauty. It was used in the preparation of medicines, ointments, and cosmetics, and Olympian athletes rubbed it on their bodies before a competition as a source of strength.

Centuries have passed, but the beneficial effects of olive oil have not faded. Today's cooking experts consider olive oil a key component of modern cooking, and nutrition experts claim its benefits over other oils. When it comes to enhancing the flavor of food, olive oil is the most effective.

So, why is it that fast-food restaurants resist the trend? Simple: olive oil is expensive and does not withstand the high temperatures produced by commercial fryers, while hydrogenated oils are cheaper and do the job just fine. As for pastries that are prepared commercially, olive oil does not have a long shelf life; it becomes rancid and changes flavor.

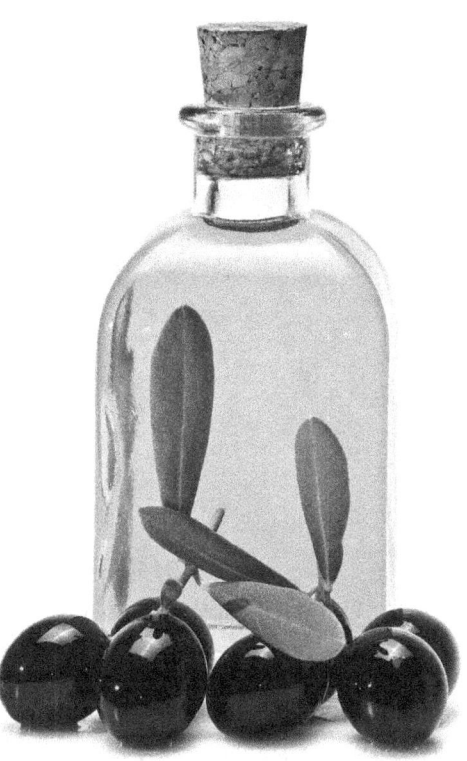

But for cooking at home, olive oil has all the advantages when it comes to flavor and health benefits. We used to reserve extra-virgin olive oil for the preparation of salad dressings and cold dishes, and we used a more processed oil for cooking. Most cooking experts today, however, agree that virgin olive oil is ideal for cooking, and since its production doesn't involve any treatments, it is clearly the one with more health advantages.

Case Scenario: Michael

Michael is a thin, healthy six-year-old who is a picky eater, but is growing normally, likes french fries so much that he requests them at every meal. Alleging they are not good for his diet, his parents try to avoid giving him french fries.

This is a common situation in many American families. Children love french fries! So, who is right, the parents or the child? The

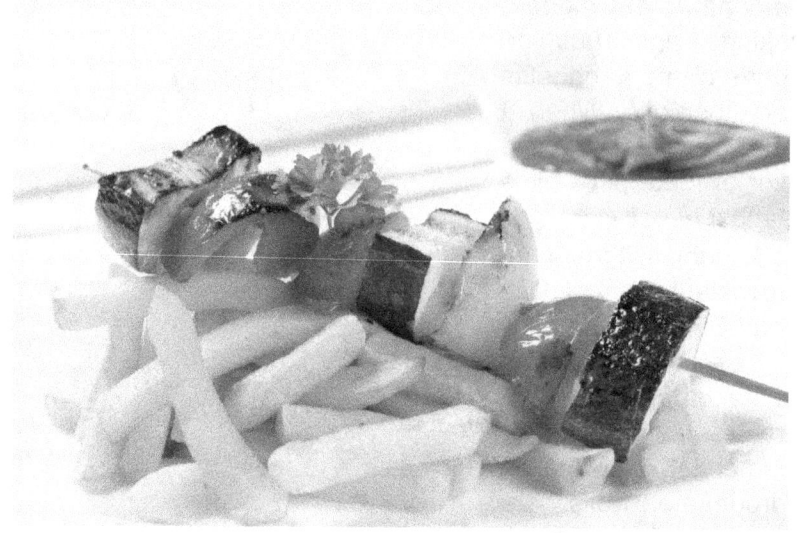

answer is tricky. Let's first look at the ingredients: we are talking about potatoes, oil, and salt. These are the only ingredients of this dish that is so loved, and yet so demonized, in our society; in many other cultures, whose populations are far skinnier than ours, a plate of french fries is typically enjoyed without any kind of guilt.

Whether or not french fries are an advisable part of any diet depends on the quality of the ingredients. If we take a couple of potatoes, fry them in a moderate amount of olive oil, and sprinkle them with a small amount of salt, then we have a perfectly accept-able companion to a protein such as meat or fish. But if, on the other hand, we use hydrogenated oil, which is going to be absorbed by the potatoes in larger amounts, we end up with a higher calorie load and a poor-quality meal.

For centuries, some Mediterranean countries—the same Mediterranean countries we often look to for examples of a healthy diet—have used olive oil to fry their food. In southern Spain, for example, they fry small fish in olive oil. This delicacy still qualifies as a healthy meal since it contains plenty of omega fatty acids from the fish and unsaturated fat from the olive oil. The end result meets our approval.

Our french fry lover should be allowed to enjoy his favorite dish after all. The only drawback of a plate of french fries made at home with good-quality oil is that it does offer a considerable amount of calories in the form of carbohydrates and fat (good fat). However, since he is healthy and thin, he doesn't have to count calories. So long as the french fries are offered in moderation and accompanied by other quality foods such as a piece of meat or fish, our picky eater is all set with a healthy and nutritious dinner.

Helpful Tips

— Olive oil should be the cooking oil of choice at home. It adds quality to meals and provides good nutrition if used in moderation.
— Since calorie counting is not advisable for most kids' (or adults') diets, using olive oil when we fry or sauté food ensures the best option for making our meals more palatable.
— We don't need to eliminate fat completely from our diets in order to lose weight and remain healthy. Moderation is the key.
— Each family needs to find the right combination of food that meets their needs. For picky eaters, including foods they like is the most effective way to get them to eat foods they don't care for.

Chapter 10

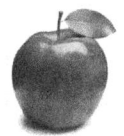 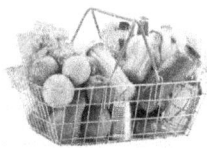 

Health and the Mediterranean Diet

Over the last century, we have witnessed a phenomenon that is going to be difficult to replicate in coming decades. With the discovery of penicillin in the 1940s, the most common causes of death shifted from infectious diseases to degenerative diseases and cancers; life expectancy increased, resulting in an older population. The increase in life expectancy brings the total number of people older than sixty years of age worldwide to more than 580 million, and this number is predicted to increase to 1 billion by the year 2020.

Are we going to be able to maintain this trend? It seems not! Our own fast-paced, modern lifestyle seems to be to blame for a possible decrease in life expectancy for future generations. This is inevitable unless we change gears, learn new ways of eating, and increase our level of daily exercise. The Mediterranean diet has the potential to be part of the solution to the increase in cardiovascular diseases in our modern society.

What is the Mediterranean diet? After all, there are more than seventeen countries surrounding the Mediterranean Sea, and each one of them has its own culinary specialties. Some common factors include the use of olive oil in the kitchen and daily consumption of fresh fruits and vegetables, combined with an active lifestyle that includes walking as the primary mode of carrying out daily errands. We should also note that meals are served in smaller portions and are accompanied by water or wine, as opposed to sodas or sweetened drinks.

In the United States, the fast-food industry produces a positive impact on the economy by creating thousands of jobs and by eliminating the need to spend time in the kitchen, thereby freeing up time for other activities or for longer working hours. The ever-increasing numbers of fast-food restaurants compete for our food dollars by offering larger meal sizes—not by a selection of quality ingredients. After all, better-quality ingredients are more expensive, and the cost would have to be passed on to the consumer; and high prices go against the whole concept of saving time and money. So, we end up with super-sized drinks, free refills, and huge servings.

Taking a look at some studies from 2009 and 2010, researchers found that adherence to a Mediterranean diet and lifestyle also decreases the risk of developing Alzheimer's disease and slows down cognitive deterioration later in life. While these studies did not point to a specific ingredient or food that would definitely lead to Alzheimer's disease, they did find that consumption of large amounts of the *wrong* foods (fats, added sugars, preservative-laden products) will prevent one from taking in the *right* foods that are protective against brain deterioration (fish, fruits, fresh vegetables, legumes); after all, only so much can be eaten in a day; choices must be made.

Granted, it is difficult to give up a lifestyle that offers convenience, saves time, and is affordable. To make a lifestyle change, my advice is to take "baby steps" in the right direction. Change just one habit per month, and by the end of the year you'll be living a healthier life. Doing something small is better than doing nothing.

Case Scenario: PK

PK is a healthy fifteen-year-old boy with a good appetite. His height has been increasing rapidly for the last three years, but so has his waistline. He likes to play video games after school, and he doesn't like to exercise at all. Even though his family lives only about one and a half miles from his school, PK's father drives him in the mornings, and his mother picks him up in the afternoons.

His parents, who are concerned about his increasing weight gain and want to help PK improve his diet, go to the school cafeteria to review what he eats for lunch. They find on offer a variety of foods, including a hot meal consisting of meat and vegetables, and they find water, milk, and chocolate milk as the choice of drinks. School officials confirm for the parents that the lunch menu does include these other choices, but that PK passes them by every day and goes directly to the pizza line. Since he has a big appetite, he opts for pizza since it is the only food that keeps him satisfied throughout the day. With his pizza, he drinks boxed juice.

Those responsible for school lunches are convinced that they do offer quality foods to students. In fact, they believe they even offer a variety of Mediterranean foods from which children may choose. That is partially true, but the healthy choices are hidden among so many unhealthy choices. In effect, the word "choice" is the problem.

If we want to take the Mediterranean culture as an example of healthy eating, then pizza should be part of the menu, right? Actually, it is very "un-Mediterranean" to trust the kids themselves to make good choices. The only way to change the school lunch is by deciding what is good, preparing it from scratch, and offering it to hungry children as the only choice. The same principle applies to the drinks offered with lunch—water or milk only.

Another "Mediterranean" change for this child would be to allow him to walk to and from school each day. If parents do not feel it is safe, they can walk with the child, making the daily walk an opportunity to exercise and share.

Helpful Tips

— Use olive oil for cooking.
— Make water the preferred beverage.
— Plan meals for a week in advance.
— If eating out, consume only half of what is served and save the rest for the next meal.
— Park at a distant point in the parking lot.
— Go for a walk in the evenings or early in the mornings.

Chapter 11

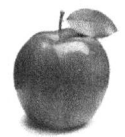 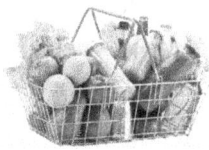 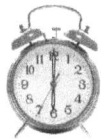

No Guilt Allowed

Have you noticed how we, as parents, tend to feel guilty about any and every negative thing that happens to our children? If they get sick, we wonder what we have done to expose them to germs; if they make a bad decision in life, we question where it is that we set the bad example or influence. Even when the defense mechanisms of our human nature make us redirect that guilt toward somebody else, deep inside we feel as if we should be able to smooth the way for our kids so they have a life perfect and free of struggles. Of course that is impossible, but that's how we feel.

Parents should not feel guilty about their children's eating habits or their own. We must replace that sensation by a feeling of energy and commitment to make changes. We need only small changes; nobody is asking you to change your entire lifestyle and forget what you have learned over decades in just one week. That would be impossible as well. Understand that it is our nature as parents to nurture and take control, to make decisions. We should learn as much as we can and then not be afraid to call problems by their name.

The Nature of Nurture

When I was growing up in Spain, my family always had a dog. The relationship we had with our animals then was very different to the one most families have these days. The dog always stayed outside, slept in a doghouse, and ate table scraps. My sister and I did play with him, but we never thought of him as part of the family. If I think back far enough, I can remember our dogs roaming outside of our backyard into the neighbor's and coming back as they pleased. Those were the times when heavy traffic was not a danger.

When my own kids were growing up, we also had a dog. I confess having no clue how to relate to the animal; but yet, we also had a couple of gerbils, an iguana, birds, and some goldfish. With three children and a full-time job, the dog was just one more thing to do and I don't clearly remember how I related to it.

A few years ago, my daughter, Natalie, now an adult, brought home a beautiful schipperke puppy. We all fell in love with him almost immediately. She set up a schedule for his care, including potty training, feeding rules, vet visits, and so on. A few months later, we adopted a sweet Yorkshire terrier puppy, who only added to the joy. Natalie continued applying her knowledge of animals to provide the best care for them, including waking up early in the morning, rain or shine, to take them for a walk and going for a second walk in the evening. She was totally in charge of animal care, and the rest of us just watched and enjoyed them.

When my daughter moved out of the house, she took the schipperke dog with her, but left little Grace, our Yorkie, with us, after we assured her we were going to take care of her the way she did. Piece of cake!

My husband and I tried keeping up with the double walk schedule, but we soon found out it was not that easy. Some mornings we are tired, and others we just forget. The reality is that Grace does not get her scheduled walks the way she used to.

As for feedings, Natalie had insisted on offering the dog a small amount of food twice a day, and putting her dish away the rest of the day, offering only water. We failed at this also. Some mornings, as I walk out of the house, I see her dish empty but still out and I assume she did not get her morning feeding; I then go and offer her more food. My husband does the same. Our lack of communication results in our leaving food out all day long, which Grace proceeds to eat without schedule. We also give her an occasional table scrap, when she looks at us with those innocent, translucent eyes while we eat. We can't resist giving her our food as we get a kick out of how happy it makes her feel.

Last week we took Grace to the veterinarian. We were surprised to learn she has gained a lot of weight, which led to a subsequent scolding by the vet, who made a list of all possible health problems the dog is facing if she continues this way, one of the main ones being a decreased life expectancy.

When we got home, feeling less proud of our ability to care for a tiny dog, we reviewed together our habits related to the care of the dog, only to realize we were making many mistakes without even noticing. We hadn't even noticed her increase in weight, yet we look at her every day!

It was an eye-opening experience for me. Here I am, advising others about the quality, quantity, and timing of the food they ingest as a way to create and maintain health, but in our care of the animal, these principles slipped right past me. It was time to humble myself and apply a dose of my own medicine.

It became clear we had issues with all three aspect of my own advice. We were making food available all day long, so the dog ate whenever she had nothing better to do. Obviously the quantity part was off, and there was no Timing at all! And in adding "human" food to the dog food she was already getting, we were creating a problem with quality. If we add to it the reduction in the frequency of walks (decrease in exercise), we clearly had a health problem in front of us.

I applaud the way our vet identified and formulated the health issues. He told us exactly what was going on, calling it "obesity" and naming the steps to follow or else. We either took his advice or our dog was going to suffer and die an early death. He was blunt and direct and didn't hide the facts, not even to make us feel better. I have to admit, I learned a lot from the visit.

As a health care provider, one of the main difficulties I encounter when it comes to obesity is to convey to the families very essential points without hurting anyone's feelings. These points are:

It is not your fault. It is nobody's fault. Leave the "blame game" to others, and just take control of the situation. It is human nature to look around for someone else to take the blame. I often hear parents mentioning grandparents as the ones to blame, because the children eat poorly when visiting them. I usually tell families not to worry so much about what children do just once in awhile but to work on what they can control: what goes on at home, on a day-to-day basis.

Yes, it is called obesity. And yes, obesity does lead to heart disease, diabetes, chronic health problems, and decreased life expectancy. Sugarcoating the truth won't take away from these fact.

Obesity is reversible. If one gets control of weight and reduces it to normal, these diseases won't necessarily be part of one's future.

This is a parenting issue. Parents should take the lead. When I am formulating a solution and giving advice to parents, I often observe how they turn to their children and say, "Do you hear the doctor? You can't drink those fruit juices you like so much." I have to redirect the focus to the parents, reminding them that they are the ones buying the juice and making it available for their kids.

Don't waste time blaming each other either. Your kids will take care of that by blaming you both in the future—if you don't do what is necessary now. If your children do go on to develop health issues as a consequence of poor eating habits in their childhood years, rest assured they are likely to tell their doctor the fault resides with the way their parents fed them. I hear this every day in my practice. Since you are going to be blamed for it anyway, don't feel bad about "laying down the law."

The Roadmap

The rubric below is designed to help you make food-related decisions on the go. First, create a brief schedule of what time and where you are going to be eating the four meals of the day: breakfast, lunch, mid-afternoon snack, and dinner. Then, if you feel hungry at any time of the day, review the following:

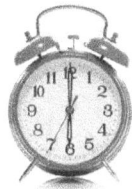

Is it time to eat?

If no – Drink a glass of water and wait one hour. After one hour, ask yourself the same question and start over again.
If yes – Select or prepare the food for that meal and ask:

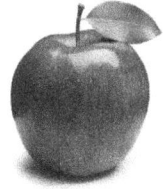

Is it quality food?

If no – Change your selection to the appropriate food, based on your knowledge.
If yes – Ask yourself:

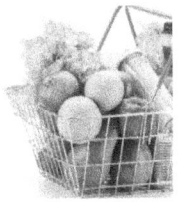

Is it the right amount of food?

If no – Decrease the amount served or change to a smaller plate.
If yes – Enjoy your meal!

Chapter 12

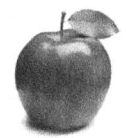 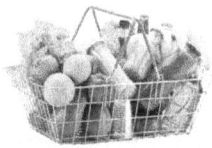 

Myth and Reality

Our times are often called "the information age." Unfortunately, some people actually believe whatever they read on the Internet, regardless of the credentials of the source. This "misinformation" can pertain to medical and health issues, as well as to many other aspects of life. I don't mean to blame misinformation only on the media or the speed of communication between people. Such myths have always existed; in fact, some older ones have resurfaced and are spreading faster than ever online.

Here I will address a few such myths in an effort to illustrate how my advice matches reality and how it contrasts with popular beliefs that are sometimes followed, albeit with the best of intentions, simply because they come from sources that we trust to be reliable.

Myth: Sugar-free or calorie-free drinks are a good option to reduce or maintain weight in children.

Reality: Since sugar-free drinks are pleasant to the taste and are preferred by children over plain water, which has no taste at all, children learn to associate the sensation of thirst with the intake of sweet-tasting fluids and, eventually, will develop a craving for sweet foods as well. Children should be offered only plain water or milk when thirsty or to accompany food intake. This is a good example of how calorie counting doesn't help much with respect to children's diets. Even foods or drinks with no calories can have an overall detrimental effect on a child.

Myth: A serving of fruit juice is equivalent to a serving of fruit.

Reality: Even if the juice is freshly squeezed at home, which most of the time it is not, a serving of fruit juice provides the body with water and sugar. That is all. When we squeeze orange juice and leave behind the pulp, we are accelerating the absorption of the sugar and contributing to dangerous shifts in our blood sugar levels that, with time, will result in insulin resistance and, ultimately, in diabetes. The reason fruits are healthy is because they provide necessary vitamins, minerals, and fiber. Their natural sugars are also healthy and necessary, but only when they are consumed as part of the whole package. Therefore, we must promote the consumption of fruits the way nature offers them to us—with all the fiber content.

Myth: Some canned pasta dishes contain a whole serving of vegetables and are a good alternative for the busy family.

Reality: Perhaps, but we are still talking about canned food. I did not make any mentions to canned food within this book, but I do advise to use food as "natural" as possible, as in "the way it comes from nature". Canned food will contain large amounts of salt, preservatives, and stabilizers to keep the food looking and smelling good. The positive effects of the serving of vegetables in the can are definitely overshadowed by the negative effects of all the other unnecessary additives. While eating canned goods during, say, a camping trip is not going to kill anyone, making them a staple at the family dinner table is not advisable.

Myth: Strawberry spreadable cream cheese over toast is an equivalent breakfast to plain cream cheese over toast.

Reality: Although toast with cream cheese is a good choice for breakfast since it provides a balance of protein and carbohydrates to start the day, when we start adding sugar, the quality of the breakfast goes down. The labels reveal that plain cream cheese contains two grams of carbohydrates per serving while the strawberry variety contains five grams. The difference is not due to the added strawberry fruit, but to the added sugar. When it comes to cheese, keep it as close as possible to nature. Some varieties contain added nuts, fruits, and honey; these options provide something new by changing the texture and adding a sparkle of flavor, but are still natural. Most varieties of strawberry cream cheese just contain sugar and added flavoring and coloring to create the illusion of strawberries.

Myth: As a children's drink, chocolate milk is equivalent to regular milk.

Reality: The only nutrient we need from milk is calcium. While chocolate milk contains the same amount of calcium as regular milk, it has more sugar. As we've established, added sugar in drinks not only means extra calories consumed; it creates a habit difficult to relinquish. The best option is not to start what we are going to have a difficult time stopping. A good rule of thumb to guarantee the proper amount of calcium intake is to offer children milk with their meals and water in between meals. After one year of age, children should be offered milk products three times per day.

Myth: Toddlers should take a vitamin supplement every day.

Reality: Toddlers should be offered vitamin-rich foods, such as fruits and vegetables, every day. When offered balanced meals and given no other meal options, children learn to eat good food that already contains all the nutrients they need to grow, and they don't need any supplementation. The only exception to this rule should be made during times of sickness when children may not be able to ingest enough food to get the proper nutrition.

Myth: A vegetarian diet is good for children.

Reality: The *Pediatric Nutrition Handbook* describes a true vegetarian as "a person who does not eat meat, fish or fowl, or products containing these foods." It also describes the different types of eating practices engaged in by vegetarians and divides them into several groups:

— *Lacto-ovo* vegetarians eat grains, fruits, vegetables, legumes, seeds, nuts, and also dairy products and eggs. They exclude meats, fish, and fowl.
— *Lacto* vegetarians don't eat eggs, but they include milk products.
— *Vegan* or total vegetarians exclude dairy products as well.

Although it is difficult to make an assessment based solely on a general description, these restrictive diets are not generally recommended for children. While it is clear that a well-balanced, planned vegetarian diet is lower in cholesterol and saturated fats, it is also deficient in vitamin B-12. Vitamin B, which is necessary for brain development and involved in many other bodily functions, is present in meats and animal products. Even with diets of legumes and other protein-containing foods, supplements are required to achieve recommended levels of vitamin B. A vegetarian diet, especially a vegan diet, also tends to contain lower amounts of zinc, calcium, and vitamin D.

It is also true that vegetarians have a decreased incidence of coronary artery disease, hypertension, and colon cancer due to the large amounts of fruits and vegetables they consume. But when researchers look at true vegetarians, they are compiling the outcome of a vegetarian lifestyle rather than the results of the diet alone. Vegetarians tend to have an increased abstinence from alcohol or they consume it in small amounts; they also tend to refrain from smoking, and they engage in more physical activity. Most true vegetarians choose this kind of diet as part of religious, ethical, or social influences, and the whole package produces healthier outcomes.

It is very different when an adolescent decides to become "vegan" because of a social trend or for weight control. Some teenagers have described to me their new vegetarian diet as one consisting of daily frozen pizza, candy bars, and sodas. While the individual components of their dietary change may meet the defined criteria, we all know that such a diet is not going to provide for the nutritional needs of their growing bodies.

The vegan food guide pyramid includes the following recommendations: six to eleven servings of grains, three or more servings of vegetables, three or more servings of fruits, six to eight servings of fortified soymilk or alternatives, two to three servings of beans. It also mentions requirements for other essentials such as supplements of omega-3 fatty acids, vitamin B-12, and vitamin D. Realizing that these recommendations are guidelines only, the truth is that, during infancy and adolescence, the amount of food required to meet the needs of the body, in energy and nutrients, may be larger than the capacity of the stomach to hold it, or it may entail multiple feedings throughout the day.

While I am respectful of different culinary traditions, I remain faithful to variety when it comes to food. Some animal species are destined to eat only grass and vegetables, and nature provided them with the right set of teeth to handle just grass and vegetables. Other animals eat only meat, and their teeth are constructed to process only meat. Human teeth, on the other hand, are designed to chew both. Nature gave us the tools to digest both vegetable products and meats, so my advice is to use the tools as nature intended.

Myth: Liquid meals, or nutritional drinks, are a good option for providing supplemental nutrition to picky eaters.

Reality: Commercial liquid meals, or nutritional drinks, are a good option for a child who is sick or unable, or unwilling, to eat. These drinks provide calories and fluids, both needed to fight infection and help the immune system. However, I don't recommend them for a healthy child—even for a picky one. Children should be trained to eat real food. When we restrict the options to only healthy foods, even a picky eater will eat, albeit perhaps in smaller portions. Giving a child calories in liquid form will only decrease or eliminate any appetite for other foods. Moreover, offering an older child a liquid meal is the equivalent of regressing to earlier stages of feeding. The solution for a picky eater lay is offering the child good quality food at scheduled times.

Part III

The
Step Up Diet

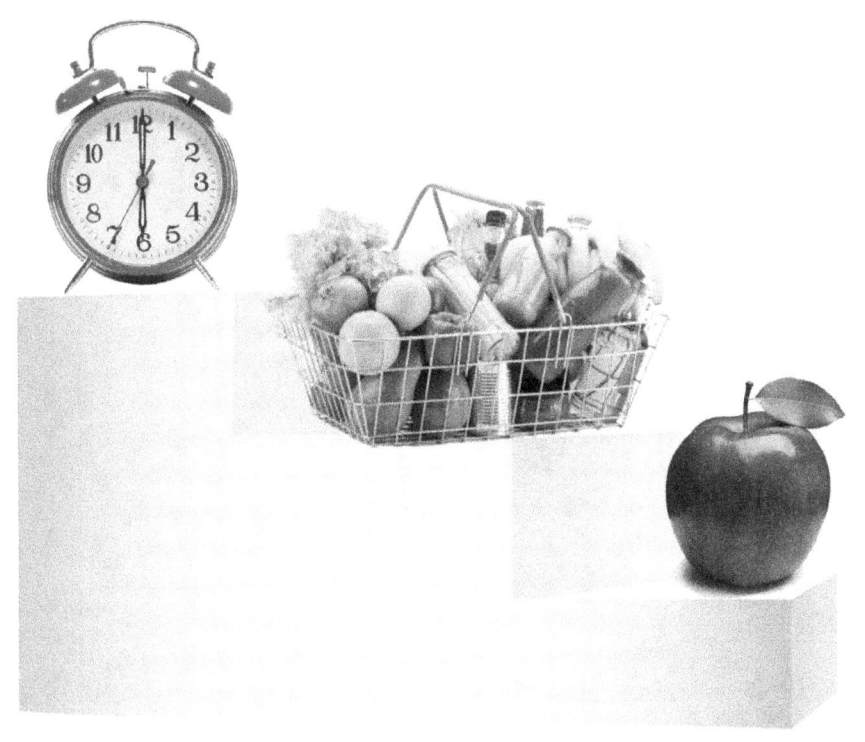

Chapter 13

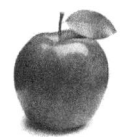 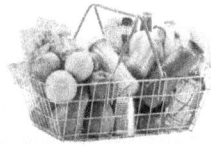 

The Step Up Diet

Unlike some diet programs, this one is not going to promise weight loss, although weight loss will occur if the body needs it. Our objective here is to achieve balance in the quality, quantity, and timing of food consumption, as discussed earlier in this book.

In order to get there, we are going to break the day into three different segments, or "steps," and start by paying special attention to each segment, one at a time, until we attain the target.

A few years ago, due to my congenital back problems, a physical therapist recommended yoga for me. I bought a DVD and started learning at home, only to set it aside after a few weeks. I didn't feel the benefits and it was boring. About one year ago, I decided to give it another try, but this time I attended yoga classes taught by a very good instructor who made me understand the purpose of all those stretches and exercises. I came to comprehend how it really works, and although I am not certain of getting it exactly right, it now works for me. Yoga teaches the body a series of poses that, when held for a few seconds, the body reads as comfortable and right. Later, during daily activities, the body tries to reproduce those motions. I observe that I now maintain a better posture and my back pain is under control. I am never going to correct my back defect, but my brain reads and recognizes what feels good and what doesn't, and it directs me toward the correct posture without my awareness.

Likewise, by training us, step-by-step, to experience what it is like to eat the right way, the Step Up Diet teaches the body and the brain to recognize what types of food are healthy to eat, and to establish a healthy eating schedule. By focusing on one step—one segment of the day—at a time, the ultimate goal becomes less overwhelming and more manageable.

Let's start by looking again at the question of body mass index (BMI). Using the formula and tables in chapter 8, measure your BMI and the BMI of each family member. If an individual's BMI is above the 85th percentile, a change is in order. On the one hand, it may be possible to achieve weight loss by adhering to a very restrictive diet for a few weeks, but the results often don't last; after some time, you're likely to be back at square one. Why? Some diets are so restrictive that they don't supply enough nutrients to keep a body going. In other words, the body and the brain do not learn anything from them. It is willpower alone making the difference. Since the body is lacking nutrition during the period of dieting, once the diet is over, the body is going to regain what was lost, and possibly more.

If, on the other hand, your BMI is on target, and this is the case for the whole family, think about the next question. Based on reading thus far, are your family's current eating habits the ones to be passed down from generation to generation?

And one final question to ask before embarking on the Step Up Diet: inquire about your family history. Is there a history of diabetes, heart disease, high blood pressure. ,or colon cancer in your family? Even a person who is not obese may have a genetic predisposition toward a disease, and if so, that may affect that person's children as well.

It is sad to recognize that the United States is the richest country in the world, yet we feed our children foods that other cultures won't touch. Moreover, we often deprive our children from knowing and becoming familiar with food the way it is presented by nature, even though the word "natural" is ubiquitous in the supermarket, and is one of the "best-selling" words in advertising.

As a pediatrician, I knew I had to do something when, several years ago, my family visited Italy, and I ordered a pizza for my then ten-year-old son, who loves pizza. Although if he had his wishes he would eat pizza every day of his life, he pushed aside a perfectly good pizza covered with natural tomatoes and other fresh vegetables. It was creating such a wonderful aroma all around that even I, who don't care much for pizza, reached for a slice. I suddenly understood what had been staring me in the face for a long time. We, in America, adopt cuisines from all over the world, transform them into a fast version with cheaper, poor-quality ingredients, add enough flavor enhancers to appeal to our taste buds, and then feed them to our children who don't know any better. They, in turn, become adults who don't know any better, and so it goes. It is for the same reason that our children drink all the fruit juice they can get their hands on but refuse to eat fruit. They like orange juice, but they won't touch an orange. Something is very wrong with this picture, and it brings a host of consequences with it.

It is difficult to create a meal schedule that accommodates our hectic American lives. Some of us get up very early and thus make the excuse that there's not enough time to prepare a healthy breakfast. Some schools offer lunch at odd times of the day (to accommodate huge student populations), thus creating a long gap between lunch and after-school snack and making it even more important that young people eat something extra before the typical dinner time. A habit that some families have that may need to change is eating dinner as early as 5 P.M. This leaves too much time after dinner for children to become hungry again before bedtime. A few weeks ago, I was evaluating a family's eating habits, and I realized they were eating three meals within a five-hour span of time: they had lunch at noon, a snack at 3 p.m., and dinner at 5 p.m. In the Step Up Diet, we are going to analyze the timing of your family meals, with the goal of scheduling four meals a day, each separated by at least three to four hours.

This diet is intended for the whole family; thus you should try to create a schedule where most meals can be shared by the entire family. It is important to eat together and to eat the same food. For one thing, it is less expensive than cooking à la carte. It also presents the only opportunity parents have to teach children good eating habits. Parents must be the experts in nutrition when it comes to our children. Their adult health depends, in large part, on what we teach them at home. Do they really have a chance of learning good eating habits at school? Take another look at the school lunch menu. You don't need to be a nutrition expert to know it is lacking.

Let's not fight with our children during mealtime. If the food offered doesn't agree with everyone, allow those who disagree to wait until the next meal. It only means they are not hungry enough, and it is perfectly fine not to eat much when not hungry.

Like with any meal plan, this one is intended for healthy individuals. Consult with your doctor before engaging in any dietary changes.

Who can use this diet plan? The answer is easy: everyone. If after calculating your BMI you find out you need to lose a few pounds while teaching your body healthy habits, you can use the following steps until reaching your level of comfort. Even if you stay at Step 1 for a while, you are going to see results. The higher up you go, the more you are going to benefit from the whole plan. But I do realize that cooking at home is not for everyone; some people travel constantly and have less control over their meals. If that describes you, then just begin by following the QQT rules and Roadmap and stay at Steps 1 and 2. Families with small children and a stay-at-home parent may find the recipes helpful and decide to use the entire diet as a guide for meal preparation.

Even families with no history of obesity and those who don't suffer from obesity can pick up some life-changing advice, since obese people are not the only ones predisposed to disease.

Step 1

The first step is very simple and easy, and it sets the stage for the three steps that follow. Do the following for two consecutive weeks:

— Eat only four times a day: breakfast, lunch, mid-afternoon snack, and dinner.
— Drink only milk or water with your meals and water only in between meals.

To put this simple plan into practice, follow the Roadmap explained earlier (see chapter 11) and repeated below. Remember that although it may be simple, it will require effort on your part if you are used to snacking constantly.

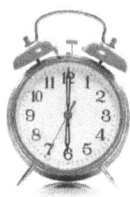

Is it time to eat?

If no – Drink a glass of water and wait one hour. After one hour, ask yourself the same question and start over again.
If yes – Select or prepare the food for that meal and ask:

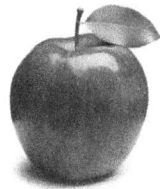

Is it quality food?

If no – Change your selection to the appropriate food, based on your knowledge.
If yes – Ask yourself:

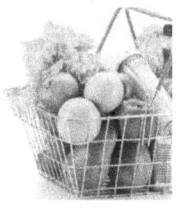

Is it the right amount of food?

If no – Decrease the amount served or change to a smaller plate.
If yes – Enjoy your meal!

Parents should monitor the snacking habits of their children and help them by eliminating sodas, chips, and sugary snacks from the house and grocery list. It is not fair to ask somebody to eliminate a habit while looking at the culprit sitting inside the pantry.

Step 2

Once you have mastered the Roadmap and established the habit of eating only four particular meals a day, proceed to Step 2. The next three steps (2–4) each focus on a different segment of the day. For each segment, I will set forth recommendations of what to eat for that period's meal.

The first segment we are going to work on is between lunchtime and dinnertime. Although it includes only one small meal, a snack, this segment is of the utmost importance, because it covers such a long stretch of time. Let's do the math: for a child or an adult who sleeps eight to nine hours per night, say from 10 P.M. to 7 A.M., the hours between lunch (at noon) and dinner (at 7 P.M.) represent almost half or the waking day. For this reason, we start with this crucial afternoon/evening segment, rather than the take up of the day's meals in chronological order.

This part of the day is important for all cultures that treasure food and good nutrition, as it used to be for ours as well. It was not too long ago that parents used to insist that their children not eat before dinner, in order not to spoil their appetites. Nowadays, with our hectic lives of after-school activities, sports events and functions to attend, we deem it acceptable to eat in the car, on the go, pretty much grabbing anything from anywhere. Sometimes, there is no real meal to be called dinner anymore. The on-the-go snack is dinner for many families. I recognize the value of sports and activities—don't get me wrong. However, if the purpose of those activities is to enrich the mind and the body, how good is it to feed the body crap (pardon me) in the process? Shouldn't we be trying to find a balance?

We are now ready for Step 2: **eat one piece of fruit and drink a glass of milk between three and four o'clock in the afternoon.**

**Here are the advantages and caveats
of this very important step:**

Fresh fruit daily: Throughout this book, we have insisted on the keys of quality, quantity, and timing as a guideline to our nutrition habits. By offering a piece of fresh fruit every day, we create the habit of eating "natural," quality food. We also take care of timing, because we are going to make sure there is no food consumption before (since lunch) or after the snack, until dinner time, which should be no earlier than 7 PM. The quantity is also loosely specified. The fruit can be large or small, and grapes, for example, can be measured into half-cup or cup servings, depending on the age of the individual.

Milk with a snack: One glass of milk given as part of a snack takes care of one-third of the daily calcium requirements at one time.

10 days of success: It can take at least two weeks of daily attempts to accomplish ten consecutive days of success, which is our goal. If you start out and, for whatever reason, miss one day, start over again until you achieve ten consecutive days of complete success. Success means the food consumed is that which is indicated for this step, and is the only food consumed during the specified period of time. That means no food while doing homework, checking e-mail, reading a book, or driving home from football practice. You can of course continue to engage in all those enjoyable activities, but without adding food or drinks (other than water) to them. If the feeling of hunger is very strong during this segment, you can drink some water or bring up the next meal, dinner, an hour earlier if you really can't wait. Drinking water becomes more important if you are engaging in exercise during this time of the day.

Cravings: During the first few days, you will be more aware of all those moments of craving a snack, if you are a child, or a cup of coffee in the case of adults. The brain, however, is going to be able to identify them as cravings for comfort food and allow them to pass. After at least ten consecutive days of success, the brain will cease craving the unneeded food, and your favorite activities will remain enjoyable even without food.

Planning: We adults make conscious choices on a daily basis; once we understand the need for a change, we are able to make the effort needed to accomplish it. Children, on the other hand, are more likely to succumb to their habits than adults are. It is up to us, the parents, to make this step a success. Don't fight over it; just have the snack of fruit and milk ready when your child returns from school. Planning ahead is more likely to produce successful results. Consult your daily schedule and plan when and where eating the snack is going to take place. If at 4 PM you are driving your child home from athletic practice, have the fruit and milk with you and offer it to your child before you drive home, or wait until you get home. Whatever you decide will be right, since you know your family and your schedule best.

Reward success: After ten consecutive days of success, you are not only ready to move to the next step, but you are also entitled to a prize! In order to keep track of your progress you can use a calendar where you are going to check off the days that you are successful. After ten marks, give yourself a pat on the back and a prize. The prize is not for the child, but for the parent, the real hero here who has succeeded in pulling through a stretch of ten consecutive days of nagging and complaints. If you are a parent, you know there are going to be some complaints, and you are going to respond to those with a big smile on your face and and "I love you." Then, move on with your plan. Your prize can be anything from a mani-pedi (manicure-pedicure) to a trip to your favorite clothing store, or a walk in the park. You deserve it and you should have it. You may encourage your child's participation by offering a small treat—something that does not involve food, or by making it into a game where siblings compete for success, and they all receive a small prize at the end for participating.

Craving healthy habits: The good news is that, after ten days of success (which might take two weeks or more of trying), your body, or your child's body, is going to crave this healthy habit and reject unhealthy ones. We are not yet talking about dinner, which I treat last (Step 4). However, you are going to notice a bigger interest in food at dinnertime after mastering this very important Step 2.

Good for the whole family: This diet should be applied to the whole family, because good eating habits are learned at home and transmitted from parents to children. It would be unrealistic for only the children or only the parents to follow this plan. The parents create the rules, based on the advice learned here, and every member of the family follows them.

Be honest with yourself: Any activity involves its ups and downs. You, as an adult, know this from experience. Recognize and accept the down moments you are going to have, and be ready to move through them. That is all part of a mental attitude that is going to be crucial in achieving the end goal. Only those who persevere are going to be successful, and this can be applied to any aspect of life. For example, how many résumés do you need to send out in order to get a job offer? Where do you want to be in life? More important, where do you want your children to be in life?

Clean out the pantry: One of the main challenges you are going to encounter resides in your pantry. If children have within eyesight and reach a large variety of snacks, it is going to be next to impossible to keep them away from those snacks. At one point or another, they are going to pay a visit to the kitchen and reach for some chips, a candy bar, or a sugary drink—if they are anywhere to be found. This program is not going to be effective until you clear your pantry of all sweets, candy, juices, chips, and any other traditional snacks.

The Perfect Snack For Toddlers

An idea for a mid-afternoon snack for a toddler is a blend of one-half to a whole banana, the juice from a freshly squeezed orange, and a half to a whole graham cracker, mixed together in a blender or food processor. This is a snack that has been fed to toddlers in some European countries for decades—one that anybody from that part of the world would remember eating.

Even today, if visiting a typical park in Spain or Italy, you will see small children running around playing with each other and, when a mother gives the signal, her child will come to her and be given a container with this ready-made healthy "treat," the only snack offered between lunch and dinner, together with a glass of milk.

This book offers additional options for snacks in chapter 17 in an effort to add variety and introduce children to other foods. But, in order to get the body and mind ready, it is important to start by creating an easy-to-follow routine.

Step 3

The segment of the day from breakfast to lunch time includes only one meal: breakfast. This segment begins when you and your children wake up in the morning and continues up to lunchtime. We are not going to discuss lunch as a particular part of the Step Up Diet, since most of us eat lunch outside of the home and thus, for the most part, parents have little control over that meal except for during weekends or vacations.

Step 3 concentrates on mastering the morning segment of the day and applying to it to what we learned in Steps 1 and 2. With these three steps, we will have taken care of a total of twelve hours of the day, or four-fifths of our waking hours, which takes us a long way toward accomplishing our end goal.

Some adolescents and many adults skip breakfast altogether. In my pediatric practice, I hear all kinds of reasons that people start their days on an empty stomach, from lack of appetite to early-morning sports practice. However, it is possible to plan and fit breakfast into any family schedule. Some serious athletes practice very early in the morning and need to eat this meal right after practice, before starting the school day. Others may have a long morning bus ride, and thus benefit from eating breakfast after they arrive at school. It may take some thinking and planning, but it is always possible.

Breakfast should include some protein. The typical quick and easy-to-prepare breakfast includes carbohydrates from a toaster pastry and some juice. We are going to modify it to include more "natural" and nutritious ingredients. You can choose and alternate between three breakfast choices described below until having breakfast becomes a routine. Once your family is used to the change, you can go to the "One-Week Sample Menu" in Chapter 14 for other choices, or to "Recipes" in Chapter 17 for even more options.

Choice A
ham-and-cheese roll-up
apple
milk

Choice B
whole wheat toast with cream cheese
banana
milk

Choice C
hard-boiled egg
grapes (½ cup)
milk

When selecting deli meat, always choose that which is freshly cut at the deli rather than the packaged variety because the former usually contains fewer preservatives. You can also ask for the "low-nitrate" choices. In order to introduce more variety, offer other deli meats, such as turkey or chicken, if you get tired of ham.

These breakfast choices are fast, require minimal preparation, and can be offered on the go. They can also be given after morning athletic practice to the child who desires to eat right before starting the school day. For adults, eating one of these breakfast options at home or after a morning workout is effective.

Adding protein to every meal increases the level of satiety. When only carbohydrates are consumed, we feel full initially, but we soon enter into the mid-morning lethargy and start craving a snack before lunch. Fresh fruit provides vitamins and fiber, which slow down the absorption of all other nutrients and prolong the sensation of being full.

While working toward achieving Step 3, continue following the mid-afternoon snack suggestions from Step 2. We are simply adding to the good habit–creating sequence.

Take note of these requirements before preparing to move on to Step 3:

You need **two weeks of success** with Step 2 (while still following Step 1).

While you can't make your child eat what you offer, you can **require that he or she eats some of the food offered**, even if the child doesn't finish all of it.

By maintaining that the periods of time between breakfast and lunch, between lunch and snack, and between snack and dinner are free of food, we are going to learn something about our bodies: **the body adapts to take advantage of food when it is available.** By keeping two- to four-hour time spans food-free for a child, he or she will be hungry by the time food is offered. This is a circumstance even picky eaters respond to. When we are hungry, we tend to eat the food given to us, even if it is not our first choice of ingredients. For example, if you are already implementing Step 1, and you are offering dinner at 7 p.m. with no other meals after, you can be sure your child will eventually start eating breakfast in the mornings. By the same token, keeping the afternoons free of food, other than the snack mentioned in Step 2, ensures a hungry participant at dinnertime.

After successfully completing Steps 1, 2, and 3, both children and adults are ready for a treat that does not involve food. At this point, you may be ready for another mani-pedi, or even a deep-tissue massage, to relax after all those times when you had to bite your tongue and turn around while pretending not to hear the comments your new food rules have provoked. Remember, parenting is not a popularity contest. (You can't get "voted off the island"!) Enforcing dietary changes is hard work and will likely place you on the bad-guy list before bringing about any positive results. For that reason, you are going to be the one providing prizes to yourself for your success. Your kids may not even recognize your efforts until they have children of their own or until later in life, when they see their friends struggling with morbid obesity while being forced to learn these simple rules as adults. It always amazes me how ready we all are to blame our parents for every habit we acquire. When I talk to parents in my practice, they blame their lack of knowledge about good habits on their own parents. I hear comments like, "My parents never cooked good food for us kids," and "My parents allowed us to drink juice and sodas," and even "I don't cook at home because I never ate homemade meals as a kid." They are correct when identifying the origin of their problem, and rest assured, your own kids are going to come to the same conclusion and blame you if they don't learn good habits in the home. That is a thought to keep in your mind while you listen to their complaints. Therefore, the massage is fully justified: you will have earned it.

Step 4

The segment of the day from dinner to bedtime includes only one meal: dinner. This period of time should be approximately three hours if dinner is offered at 7 p.m. Although the duration is relatively short, it is key to finishing the day on track.

By now you may have noticed the somewhat arbitrary division of the day, as well as the equal emphasis placed on the mastery of each step, regardless of how much food consumption is involved. To clarify, in the Step Up Diet each part of the day is important based not only on the value of the nutrition provided by the meal included in that segment, but also on the period of time around that particular meal—that is, the time spent not eating. In this program, what you don't eat is just as crucial as what you eat. It is of vital importance that you engage in your daily activities without including snacks or comfort foods. In our culture, being trained to not eat may be a novel concept, but it is the key to success in aiming for long-term results.

In American culture, dinnertime is when the family typically has time to prepare a more complete meal, and all family members are usually home to enjoy it. We are going to leave aside the debate as to whether this time of the day is the appropriate time to eat a large meal (in some other cultures, it is not

Keep in mind that the prior steps should be maintained during the three weeks of working through the various dinner menus. The purpose of this step is to encourage home-cooked dinners that require minimal preparation while maximizing the quality of the food.

Week One

On Sunday evening, prepare the following homemade tomato sauce that can be frozen until it is used for two different dinners of the upcoming week, Monday and Friday.

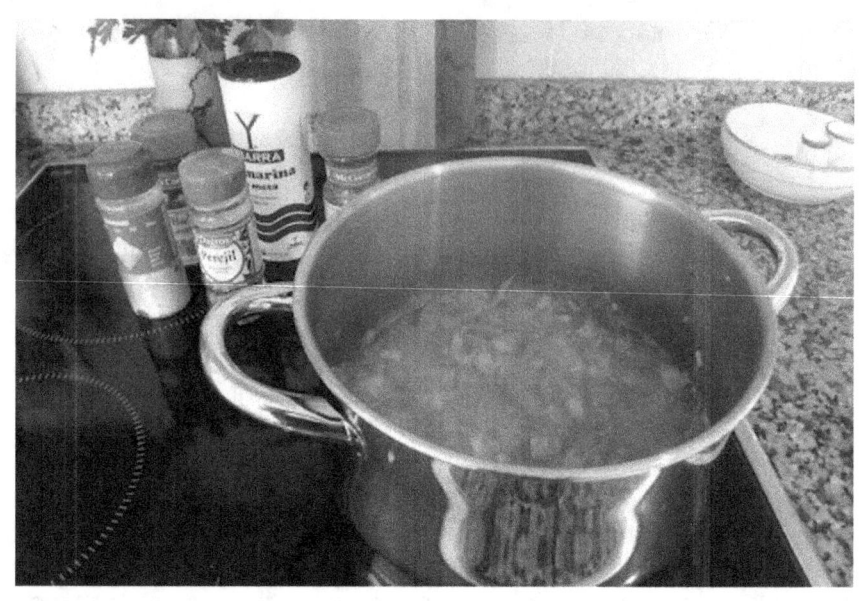

PASTA WITH HOMEMADE TOMATO SAUCE
(FOR MONDAY AND FRIDAY)

Ingredients
1 carrot
1 leek
4 large, fresh tomatoes or 1 can (29 oz.) tomato puree
½ onion
2 garlic cloves
¼ cup fresh parsley
4 tablespoons olive oil
oregano
basil
salt and pepper

Preparation
In a saucepan, heat four tablespoons of olive oil over medium heat. Cut the onion, garlic, leek, fresh parsley, and carrot into small pieces, and heat it in the oil for about five minutes. Add the tomato puree or the fresh tomatoes (peeled and cut). Cook on low heat for

about 30 minutes more. Remove from heat, and mix, using a hand blender, until all the ingredients form a sauce of uniform consistency. Add the dried oregano, basil, salt, and pepper, to taste, and cook over medium heat for an additional ten minutes.

On Monday night and Friday night, we are going to cook half a pound of pasta (spaghetti one day and penne pasta the other day) and will serve the defrosted tomato sauce on top of the pasta.

We are now practicing how to prepare a completely homemade, all-time favorite from natural ingredients, without preservatives.

Week Two

This week, you will again cook pasta for the same two days of the week, Monday and Friday, and make a bean soup for another two days of the week, Tuesday and Thursday. Does this sound too repetitive? Not really—if you consider that most families eat the same fast-food meals over and over again. The goal here is to learn how easy and delicious home cooking can be. All of these dishes have been kid-tested and approved. If you think your own family may not appreciate it at first, be ready to respond with the same smile you are, by now, mastering.

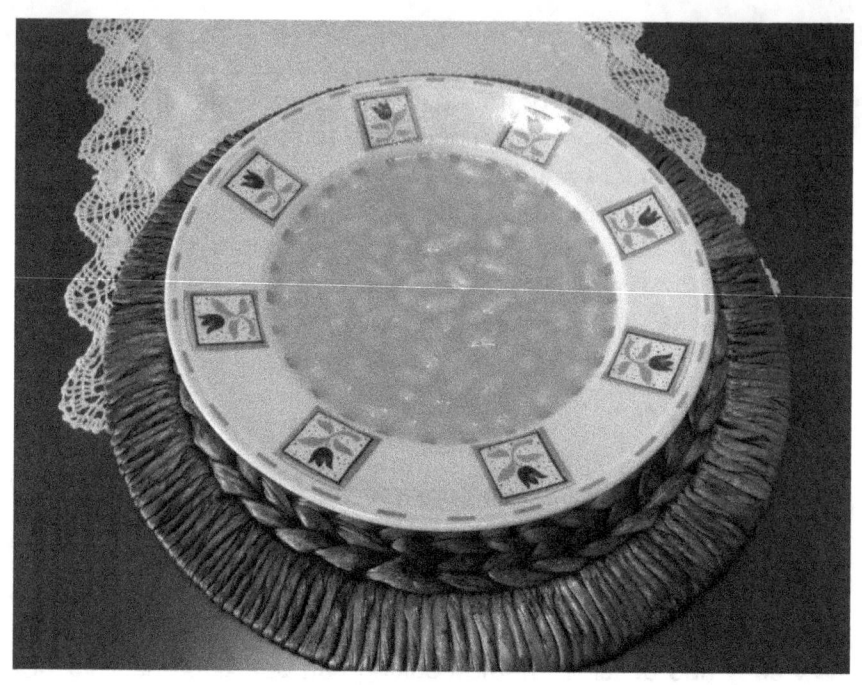

BEAN SOUP
(FOR TUESDAY AND THURSDAY)

Ingredients
½ lb. dried, white beans (or northern beans)
1 carrot
1 leek
½ onion
1 garlic clove
1 sausage (Italian, or any other kind your family likes)
2 teaspoons paprika
6 tablespoons olive oil
salt

Preparation
Soak the beans the night before. Some claim soaking eliminates a large part of the gas-creating component in legumes. In any case, it helps to speed up the cooking process.

Chop the carrot, leek, onion, and garlic into small pieces and place them in a large pot with about three tablespoons of olive oil. Cover and cook over medium heat for about eight minutes until the onions are transparent and the water is cooked out of them. Add the dried beans after they have been soaked, and then add enough cold water to cover the beans. Cook over low heat for about one and one-half hours until the beans are soft. Alternately, you may use a pressure cooker for twenty minutes, or a Crock-Pot to allow for cooking all day. Add cold water in small amounts if the beans look dry during the cooking process.

In a saucepan, add three tablespoons of olive oil. Cut the sausage into small pieces, and cook it in hot oil for about three minutes. Add the paprika to the sausage and stir. Now add the cooked, seasoned sausage to the cooked beans and stir well. Allow to cook for another ten to fifteen minutes, and it will be ready to serve.

For toddlers who might refuse to try something unfamiliar because of its color or texture, you may use a blender or a hand mixer, or just mash the beans with a fork before serving.

This recipe provides dinner for four people. You may double the ingredients and cook the entire bag of beans (1 lb.), freezing the leftovers for another day.

Week Three

You may offer this soup on Wednesday while again serving the pasta dish on Monday and Friday and the bean soup on Tuesday and Thursday. These meals combined cover the whole work week.

"Hulk Soup" is a nickname my family gave to this recipe when I used to prepare it for my picky children. I told my youngest, a fan of The Incredible Hulk, that this soup is what his favorite character eats in order to keep his strength and the green color of his body. Even though he knew it was not true, my son found my story amusing, and he ate the soup with a big smile on his face.

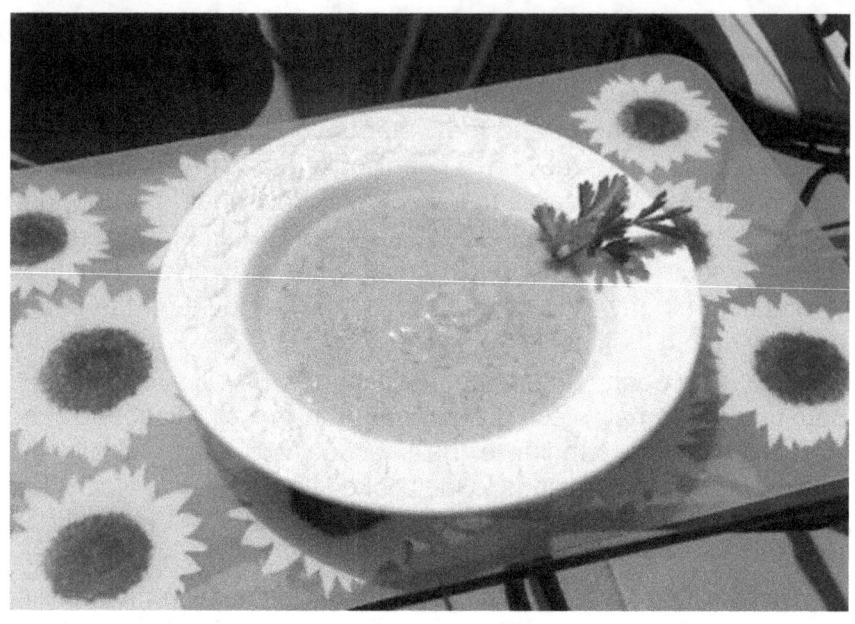

"HULK SOUP" OR VEGETABLE SOUP
(FOR WEDNESDAY)

Ingredients
3 medium zucchini
1 medium onion
3 medium potatoes
1 stalk celery
2 garlic cloves
8 oz. cream cheese
3 tablespoons olive oil
salt and pepper

Preparation
Cut the zucchini, onion, potatoes, celery, and garlic into small pieces. Place them in a pot and barely cover with water. (Since we are not draining the vegetables after cooking them, we don't want to add too much water; it will make the soup too thin.) Add three table-spoons of olive oil. Bring to a boil and cook at medium temperature until all ingredients are soft.

Remove the pot of boiling vegetables from the heat and, without draining the water, use a hand mixer to blend all ingredients into a fluid, vegetable puree. Add the cream cheese to the mixture and resume cooking on low heat until the cheese melts and mixes well with the vegetables. In order to obtain a more uniform consistency, the mixture may need to be blended again after adding the cheese. Add salt and pepper to taste.

By week three, you will have mastered a whole week of home-made dinners. For Saturday and Sunday, you are on your own, but I can assure you that you'll be eating leftovers or preparing something similar for those two days. By now, your palate and your body will be craving good food, and it will become more and more difficult to settle for less.

What about Lunch?

As noted earlier, most of us eat lunch outside of the home, which makes this meal the most difficult to control. Some kids take their lunch from home, which typically consists of a sandwich, chips, and juice. Others eat the cafeteria lunch, which offers some good choices; however, we have learned that offering choices is not necessarily conducive to teaching children good eating habits. It would be much more productive if schools would stick to one nutritious, homemade meal per day. (See chapter 18.)

If packing a lunch for your kids, you don't have many choices. Since most schools lack the ability to refrigerate or reheat food for students, taking leftovers from dinner is often impractical. The sandwich option is the most practical one. Stay away from chips, candy bars, and juice. Instead, send cheese sticks, fresh fruits, frozen yogurt, and milk or water to drink.

Even when we leave lunch out of the equation, by mastering the other meals of the day and the periods of time in between those meals, we end up with a solid foundation of quality food preferences and a healthier meal schedule.

Chapter 14

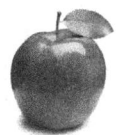 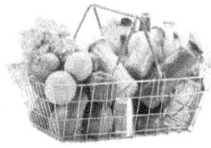 

One-Week
Sample Menu for a
Family of Four

This meal plan is not a diet; it is a menu. It is intended for healthy families who anticipate remaining healthy, but it is also suitable for those with some health issues. Most adults who have a health condition such as diabetes, high blood pressure, or high cholesterol know what they can and cannot eat. Any questions, however, should be run past a doctor. People with diabetes are particularly sensitive when eating an unbalanced meal; they rapidly see the impact in their sugar levels. This menu takes into consideration a balance of nutrients. For one whose diabetes is severe or out of control, this plan may not be suitable. Those with health problems should always follow a doctor's advice and check with a health care professional before changing any eating habits.

As mentioned in a previous chapter, people have preferred cooked food since the discovery of fire. Cooked vegetables, for example, are easier to digest than raw ones. For many reasons, I promote cooking at home. For one, the use of fresh ingredients versus canned products, chemicals, and additives is a way to improving and maintaining good health. For another, kids' eating habits are acquired from their parents, at home. Additionally, when cooking at home, we can use olive oil as our preferred cooking oil; we know that cultures that use olive oil as their primary source of fat have a decreased incidence of cardiovascular disorders. For the busy, modern family, however, cooking at home may seem like a daunting task.

I like to believe that with having a full-time pediatric practice and three children, I am one of the busiest people on earth. I can promise that it is possible to organize one's family life in a way that allows time for meal preparation. For me, Sunday is the ideal day for grocery shopping. Having a spouse with whom to share the shopping and cooking experience can make the kitchen more fun. Older children can be a big help too. Although I made this menu with the working family in mind, it can help stay-at-home parents as well. The aim is to provide a basic plan to follow that answers the "What am I going to cook tomorrow?" question.

Most of us eat breakfast and dinner at home. American families tend to eat lunch out during the week; parents grab something close to work, and kids eat at school. For that reason, I include suggestions for breakfast and dinner only, adding an afternoon, after-school snack for children. When families prepare a lunch to send to school with a child, it usually consists of a sandwich and some fruit or yogurt. Kids who eat school lunches have different choices, and we have little control over what they select. But if children learn to eat well-balanced meals at home, they will make better choices at the school's cafeteria, and eventually, when they become adults in charge of their own meals, they will continue to make healthy choices. After all, this is the goal: to expose children to a variety of good food early on in order to prepare them for an adult life of options.

As for portion size, notice that I don't address that when describing the meals. That aspect is up to the individual who serves the meal. If children or a spouse tend to overeat, serve their meals restaurant-style: decide what is appropriate and place it in front of them. If they are still hungry at the end of the meal, allow them to eat more fruit or another serving of salad. Most overeating, however, is done between meals, so the key is not just to plan the meals but for family members to eat at the table only. Don't allow children to eat while they are watching TV or using the computer. Sodas, juices, and chips are sources of empty calories and extra pounds. Therefore, don't provide them, period. If children don't eat that kind of food in the house, they won't learn to crave it later on. Deal with the picky eater in the same way; present the food and encourage eating without fighting or stress. When children are not given options, they eventually learn to enjoy good food. We are all a little different when it comes to the amount of food we need to subside. When children who only require small amounts of food are given larger amounts of their preferred foods in hopes of increasing their intake, not only are they not going to eat more; in the end, they will never learn variety in their food choices. Families with very small children may have leftovers every day and may not need to cook but every other day. Toddlers may eat only one of the foods offered for dinner; this is perfectly appropriate and will allow leftovers for the next day.

Some of the dishes on this menu include ingredients, such as saffron or Spanish pimentón, with which some people may not be familiar. Spanish pimentón adds a special taste to any dish; it can be used in sauces or with meats or fish. Saffron, which has been used widely since ancient times by Mediterranean cultures—not only in the kitchen, but also in perfumes and as a tonic with medicinal properties—gives a unique aroma to rice and fish dishes as well. I just can't imagine a kitchen without pimentón, saffron, garlic, or parsley. I am not trying to be difficult or exotic; I simply learned to cook this way, and those two ingredients are essential in a Mediterranean-style meal. Remember, I am not a chef; I am a mother, a wife, and a doctor. I go through the same struggles as others on a daily basis. I learned what I know from my mother, who learned from her mother. (Welcome to the family!)

Because of my medical training, I enjoy putting together ingredients that I know are healthy, and I always have fun in the process. After years of practicing this, I can see that my efforts are not wasted; I watch my two adult children enjoying and choosing healthy foods while I continue to struggle with a teenager. With practice, each individual will be able to introduce their own variations to a meal. That is how culinary traditions are created. As I tell parents, "Think about your kids coming home and asking you to prepare that special soup or meat they enjoy. Later, it will be your grandkids requesting your specialties." And throughout it all, have fun! Meal preparation should be a creative and relaxing time of day and can be shared by the whole family.

As mentioned previously, I suggest drinking water or milk with meals. Since children need three servings of calcium-containing food per day, I advise serving milk with the meals and water between meals. However, many dishes already contain cheese, and other milk products are also included in breakfast and snacks, and this allows for more flexibility when it comes to choosing what to drink with meals. The grocery list provided in this book does not indicate what amount of milk to buy for the week because every family is different and already knows how much is regularly consumed. Some prefer soy milk or almond milk; others choose rice milk, milk with acidophilus, low-fat/2 percent milk, or nonfat milk. It doesn't really matter. Since small children who are healthy don't need to follow a fat-free diet, whole milk is a valid option. Some parents tell me they prefer to buy only one kind of milk for the entire family; if they all enjoy low-fat milk, then low-fat milk it is.

While grocery shopping on Sunday afternoons in preparation for this menu, notice the contents of the grocery cart. They may be very different from what's in fellow shoppers' carts. While most people buy canned or prepared foods, the individual following this plan is going to have a cart loaded with fresh produce. That is a good thing. Some parents express concern about the price of the groceries required for fresh, home cooking, but I don't believe there is a big difference; those who eat unhealthy food tend to eat large quantities of it, as well as snack foods, which makes grocery bills higher. It is better to eat small portions of good food than to load up on junk. The financial benefits of healthy food are gained by having a stronger immune system, which translates into fewer trips to the doctor as well as long-term prevention of chronic disease. This is especially important for kids, because their immune systems are developing, their brains are growing, and they are acquiring habits that are going to follow them for the rest of their lives.

After all, we are what we eat. Think about that when looking at the contents of the grocery cart.

Keep in mind that this menu is the ideal, and it may be difficult to achieve immediately. Some may prefer to transition gradually into this healthier lifestyle by taking smaller steps in the beginning. It is for this purpose that I created the Step Up Diet plan. The Step Up Diet uses the same "Sample Menu" and moves gradually toward the same end goal, but rather than trying to change an entire lifestyle all at once, it aims at mastering one segment of each day at a time, and over a period of time, the desired changes are brought about.

Sample Menu for a Family of Four

Sunday

Dinner: Lentil Soup and Beef with Vegetables

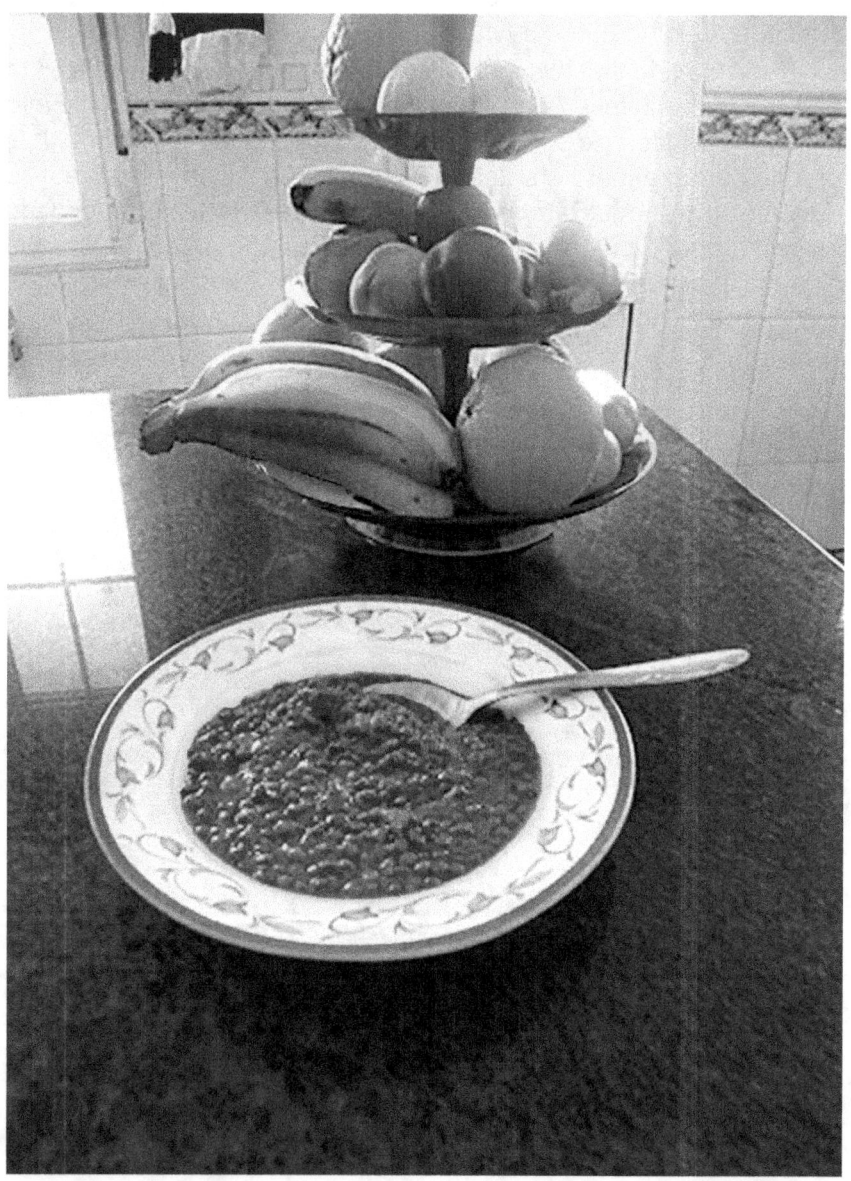

LENTIL SOUP

Ingredients
1 lb. dry lentils
2 leeks
2 medium carrots
3 garlic cloves
½ onion
11 tablespoons olive oil
2 teaspoons Spanish pimentón
2 Spanish chorizos or 2 Italian sausages

Preparation
Soak the lentils in warm water for three to four hours or overnight.

Chop the carrots, onion, leeks, and garlic into small pieces and place them in a separate pot. Add six tablespoons of olive oil and cook the vegetables over medium heat, covered, until the onions start to look transparent. Uncover.

After draining the water from the lentils, add them to the pot of sautéed vegetables. Stir for a few seconds, and add enough cold water to cover the lentils slightly. While partially covered, cook over low heat for about one hour. As the lentils cook and absorb water, you may need to add more water periodically; check them every fifteen minutes and add cold water as needed.

* Note: While the lentils are cooking, go ahead and prepare the Beef with Vegetables.

The soup will start to thicken as the cooking progresses. Remember to add water as needed. The soup shouldn't be too runny or too dry. Stir frequently to get an idea of the consistency.

When the lentils are cooked (after one to one and one-half hours), it is time to prepare the Spanish chorizo or Italian sausage to add to the soup.

Cut the Spanish chorizo or Italian sausage into very small pieces. Place five tablespoons of olive oil in a saucepan over medium heat, and add the chorizo or sausage to the oil as it begins to warm up. After three minutes and while stirring, add two teaspoons of Spanish pimentón. Allow the mixture to cook over low heat for one more minute. Add the chorizo or sausage mixture to the lentil soup, stirring constantly. Remove from heat, cover, and allow to cool for 30 minutes before serving.

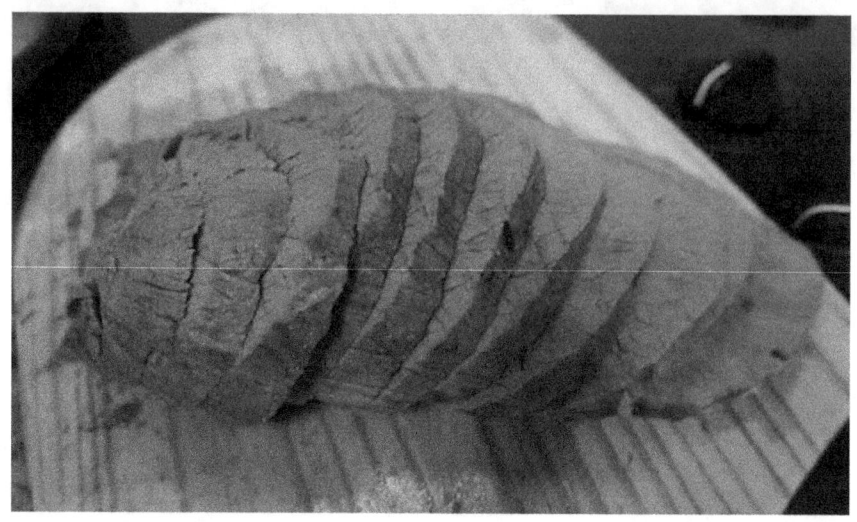

BEEF WITH VEGETABLES

Ingredients
2 lbs. beef rump roast
1 medium onion
½ green bell pepper
½ red bell pepper
2 garlic cloves
2 carrots
6 tablespoons olive oil
2 teaspoons Spanish pimentón
¼ cup white wine
1 bag frozen peas and carrots (10 oz)

Preparation
Chop the onion, carrots, garlic, red pepper, and green pepper into small pieces. Pour six tablespoons of olive oil into a pot over medium heat, and add the chopped vegetables. Place the roast on top of the vegetables, and cover for a few minutes. When the vegetables start cooking and produce a sizzling sound, cover and allow it to cook for five minutes. Turn the roast over, and allow it to cook for five more minutes.

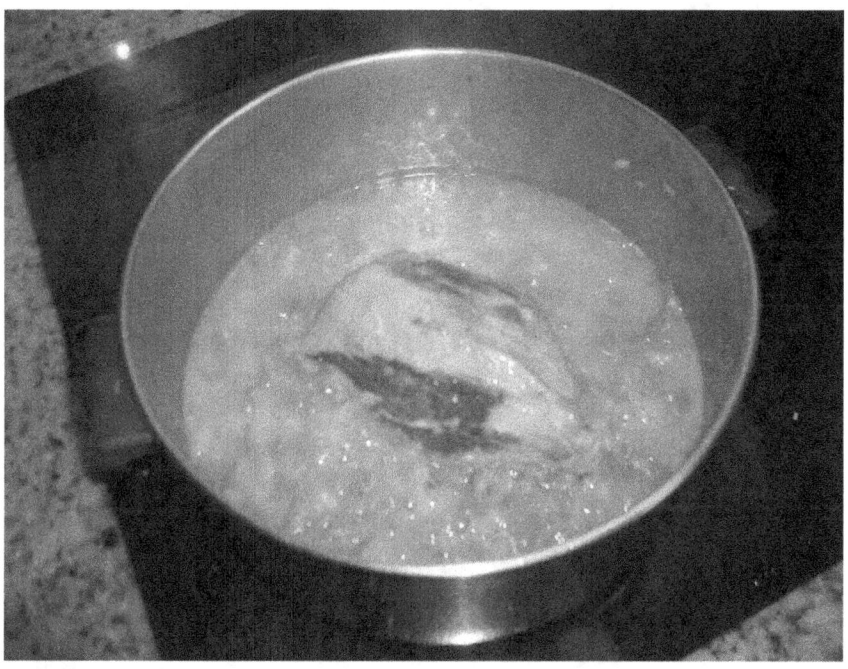

* Note: Save the unused half red pepper and half green pepper from this recipe for use in Saturday's brunch.

Once the whole roast is slightly brown all around, add enough water to cover the vegetables. Then add the white wine and cover. Allow it to cook over low heat for about 45 minutes, while turning the roast over every 15 to 20 minutes to allow it to cook evenly.

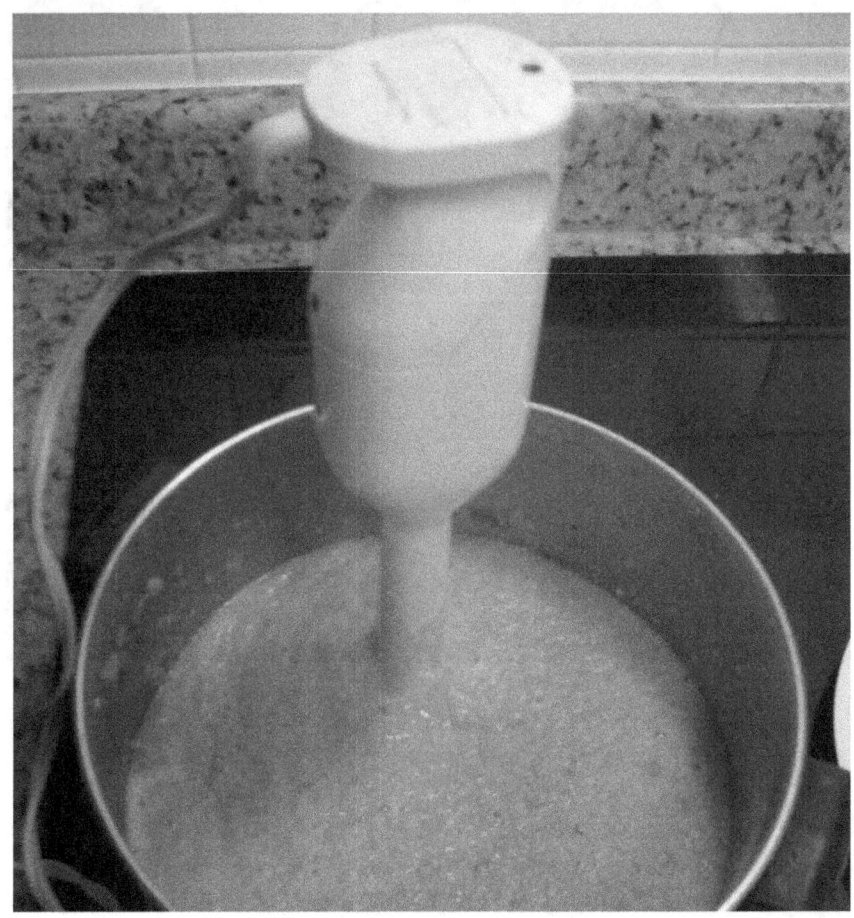

After the 45 minutes, take the roast out of the pot while leaving the vegetables inside the pot, and allow the roast to cool before cutting it. Now, using a hand-held mixer, blend together all the vegetables in the pot until they are completely pureed. Add salt and two teaspoons of Spanish pimentón, and continue cooking on low heat.

By hand, or using an electric meat cutter, cut the meat into quarter inch thick slices. Depending on how thick the roast is, some pink or bleeding at the center of the meat may be visible. This does not matter, as the roast will be cooked some more.

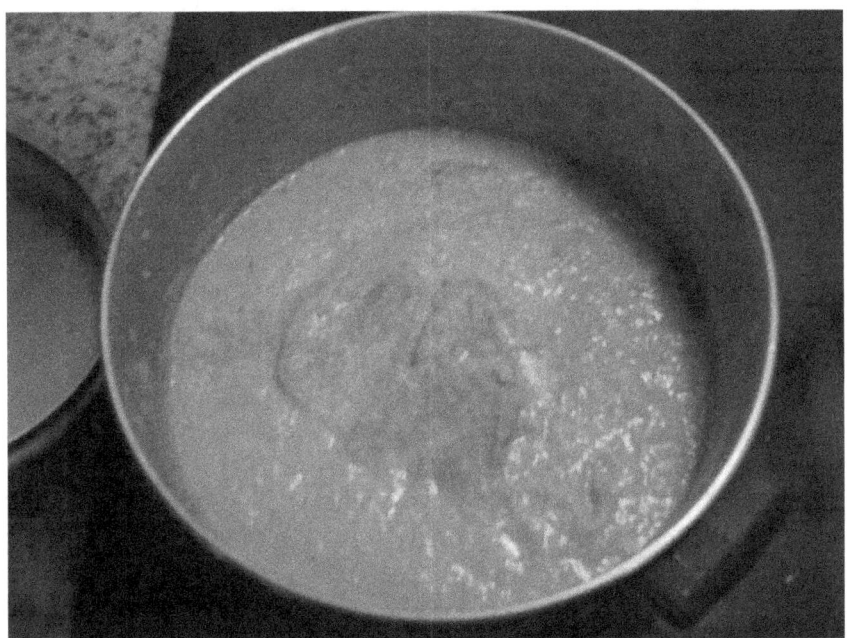

Add the sliced meat to the vegetable mixture, and then add the frozen peas and carrots, and cover. Allow it to cook on low for another 30 to 40 minutes.

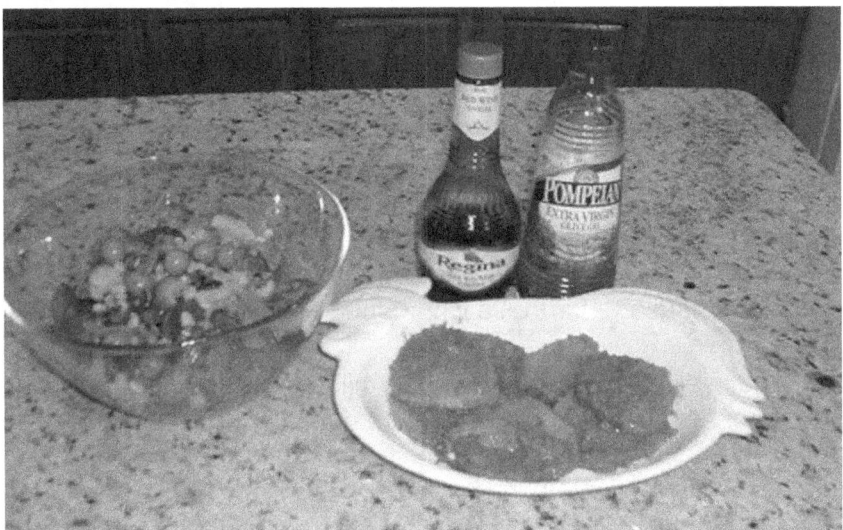

The dish is now ready. Keep it in the pot until time to serve.

* Note: This dish will suffice for two dinners: both Sunday's and Monday's. Also, spoon out approximately one cup of the sauce from the Beef with Vegetables, place it in a freezer bag, and put it in the freezer to be used on Tuesday.

Sunday Explanations

We now have a nutritious dinner: a bowl of "lentil soup," followed by "beef with vegetables." We prepare these two dishes on a Sunday afternoon because they require more time to cook and a higher level of supervision.

Because Sunday is usually a relaxing day for most families, we are going to begin our menu on a Sunday afternoon or evening. Most of us come and go from home as we share time with family. Whether we decide to go out for breakfast or to sleep-in and skip breakfast, we are going to have the time to gather the ingredients for the week simply by including a few easy steps. For working parents in particular, Sunday is the day that allows more time for strolling around the grocery store gathering ingredients for their meals. I planned the weekly grocery shopping outing for Sunday for this very reason. Once people start enjoying the whole experience, they may find, over time, that they need to visit a couple of grocery stores to find the best produce or prices.

Sunday's menu includes an ingredient that is little known to traditional American families, but is loaded with nutritional and health benefits. Lentils are legumes; they are rich in fiber and iron and they are ideal for people who need to watch their cholesterol levels or their blood sugar. Lentils allow for slower absorption of all other ingredients on the menu creating satiety and preventing overeating. Lentils are 25 percent protein; in itself, a bowl of lentils constitutes a meal.

In this recipe, we add Spanish chorizo or Italian sausage increasing the protein content of the dish. The Spanish chorizo or Italian sausage is actually an optional ingredient; while this menu is intended for healthy people, the dish can be prepared without the chorizo or sausage for those who need to decrease the fat content of their meals.

Lentils are also well tolerated by all age groups. For a toddler, a bowl of "lentil soup" is a complete meal. If a child cannot tolerate the texture of the soup, the lentils can be put through a strainer to create a more delicate puree.

The amount of lentils recommended in this recipe is more than enough for a family of four. It is difficult to generalize when it comes to the amount of the ingredients; for example, if a family of four includes two teenagers, the amount indicated in this menu may be just what is needed. If, on the other hand, the family includes two small toddlers, less "beef with vegetables" may need to be prepared since toddlers may become full with just a bowl of lentils for dinner. Most likely, there are going to be leftover lentils; they can be placed in a freezer-safe bag and frozen for future meals. For a particularly busy day when cooking is not an option, place the lentils in the refrigerator in the morning and the soup will be defrosted by dinnertime.

Our "beef with vegetables" dish is easy to prepare, although it may seem complicated at first. Just think about the amount of vegetables that can be "camouflaged" into this meal, kept away from the judging eyes of picky eaters. And because of the amount of beef and the generous quantity of vegetables added, there is enough for the next day's dinner.

* Note: Spoon out approximately one cup of the sauce from the "beef with vegetables," place it in a freezer bag and put it in the freezer to be used on Tuesday.

As a drink with meals, I always recommend serving milk to children to add calcium to the diet. Water is another option for adults. And, even after this hearty dinner, growing kids with healthy appetites may have room for an apple or a few grapes, so keep a bowl of fresh fruits in the kitchen to offer after any meal.

Monday

Breakfast

HAM AND CHEESE ROLL-UP WITH FRESH BLUEBERRIES

Ingredients
1 slice deli ham
1 slice cheese
½ cup fresh blueberries
1 glass milk

Preparation
Roll up the ham and cheese and accompany with fresh blueberries.

Pour one glass of milk. (A glass of calcium-fortified orange juice could substitute for the milk if desired.)

Afternoon Snack

PEANUT BUTTER FAVORITE

Ingredients
1–2 celery sticks
peanut butter (4 tablespoons)
1 apple

Preparation
Spread the peanut butter on the celery sticks and/or on the apple.

Dinner: Beef with Vegetables and Salad

BEEF WITH VEGETABLES AND SALAD

* Note: Beef with Vegetables was prepared on Sunday. Just add a salad.

Salad Ingredients
½ head lettuce
1 tomato
1 handful fresh blueberries
¼ bag spinach
olive oil
vinegar

Preparation
Chop produce and mix together. Add a splash of oil and vinegar.

* Note: Save the remaining ¾ bag of spinach for Thursday's dinner.

Monday's Explanations

Today's breakfast includes some protein provided by the ham and cheese, while fiber, extra vitamins, and antioxidants come from the blueberries. Milk adds the calcium children need for bone health.

The afternoon snack includes peanut butter, one of kids' favorites, while providing the fiber and vitamins contained in the celery and apple.

Dinner is already prepared since we made enough Beef with Vegetables the day before. The amount of beef per person varies; small children may need their meat processed to make smaller bites. Since the ground vegetables used in the preparation of the meat provide enough sauce, it makes for a smooth dish that is suitable for small children.

The salad part of the meal may contain various vegetables. This salad includes lettuce, tomatoes, fresh spinach, and a handful of blueberries. For dressing, we can add some salt, olive oil, and a favorite variety of vinegar.

Tuesday

Breakfast: Cheese Toast and Banana

Ingredients
1 banana
1 slice whole wheat toast
1 slice cheese
1 glass milk

Preparation
Melt one slice of cheese over a slice of whole wheat bread and accompany with a banana and a glass of milk.

Afternoon Snack: Yogurt and Apple

Ingredients
1 yogurt
1 apple
Preparation
Choose one yogurt and accompany with an apple. The best yogurt is, naturally, the plain one. For those not used to the sour taste of fresh plain yogurt I recommend adding two teaspoons of honey.

Dinner: Pasta with Parmesan Cheese and Meat Sauce, Cucumber and Tomato Salad

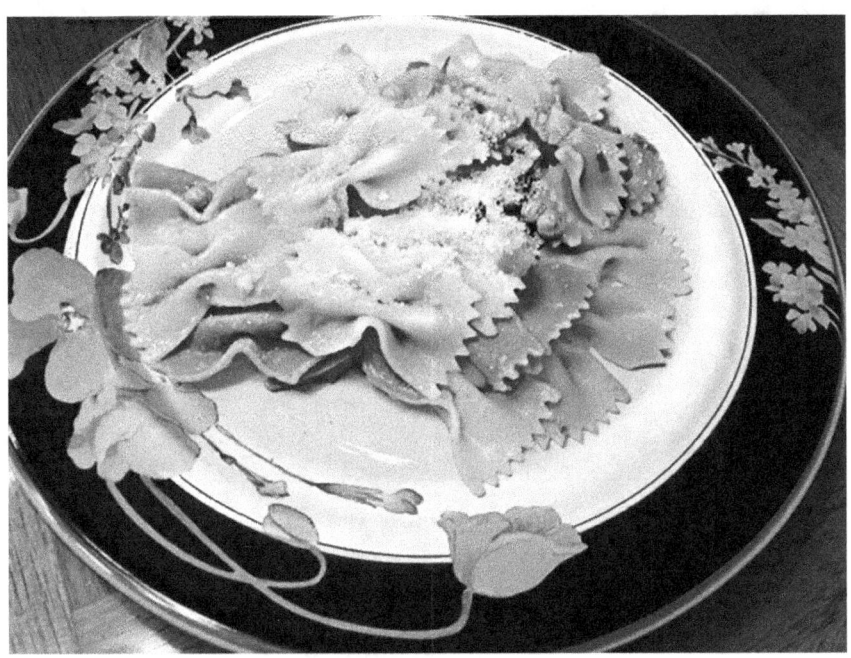

PASTA WITH PARMESAN CHEESE AND MEAT SAUCE

Ingredients
¾ lb. multi-color bowtie pasta
1 cup meat sauce
2 tablespoons grated Parmesan cheese

Preparation
Defrost meat sauce *(*note: from Beef with Vegetables cooked on Sunday)* in refrigerator.

Cook the multi-color bowtie pasta with a pinch of salt in abundant boiling water for about 15 minutes or until tender. Drain and set aside.

Warm the defrosted meat sauce, and add it to the pasta along with about two tablespoons of grated Parmesan cheese. (If any meat from the Beef with Vegetables remains, cut it into small pieces and add them to the pasta as well.)

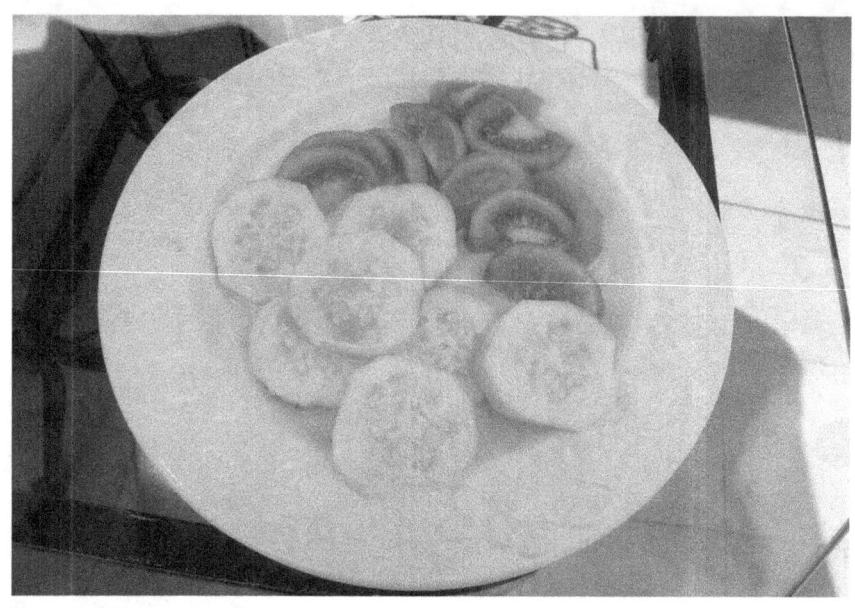

CUCUMBER AND TOMATO SALAD

Ingredients
1 cucumber
1 tomato
dill weed
olive oil
vinegar

Preparation
Chop the cucumber and tomatoes and add a small amount of olive oil and vinegar. Add dry dill weed to taste.

Tuesday's Explanations

Today's breakfast begins the day with calcium-containing milk and cheese. The cheese also supplies protein, while extra fiber is provided by the whole wheat bread and banana.

A yogurt and apple for the afternoon is a simple way to provide nutrients without interfering with dinner.

Dinner includes pasta, which is typically well liked by young and old, mixed with a meat sauce that has been carried over from the Beef with Vegetables and grated Parmesan cheese. As noted, any leftover meat from the Beef with Vegetables dish may be cut into small pieces and added to the pasta as desired.

As for the salad, cucumber and tomatoes add fiber, flavor, and texture to the meal.

Wednesday

Breakfast: Egg with Toast

Ingredients
1 hard-boiled egg
1 slice whole wheat toast
1 glass milk
Preparation
Serve hard-boiled egg and whole wheat toast. Pour one glass of milk.

*`Note: Egg can be boiled and peeled the night before.

Afternoon Snack:
Chopped Banana and Apple Salad

Ingredients
1 banana
1 apple
Preparation
Chop banana and apple into bite-size pieces and mix together.

Dinner: "Hulk" Soup (Vegetable Soup) and Breaded Pork Cutlets

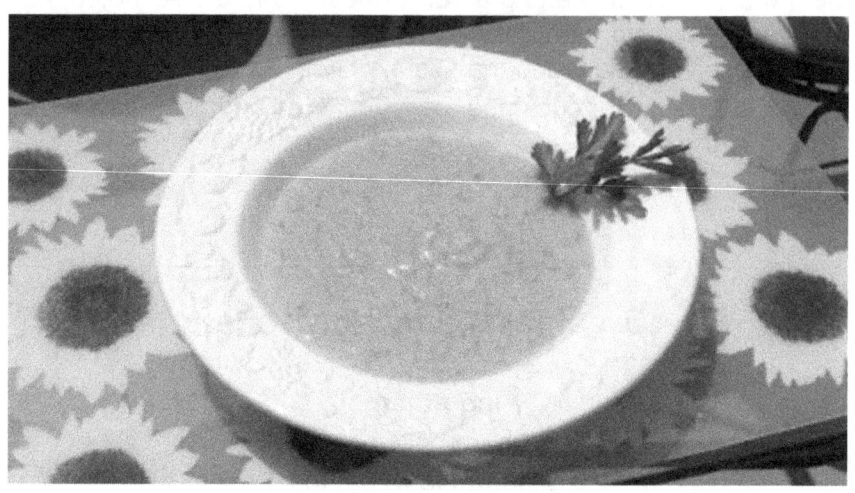

"HULK" SOUP

Ingredients
3 medium zucchini
1 medium onion
3 medium potatoes
1 stalk celery
2 garlic cloves
8 oz. cream cheese
3 tablespoons olive oil
salt and pepper

Preparation
Cut the zucchini, onion, potatoes, celery, and garlic into small pieces. Place them in a pot, and barely cover with water. (Since we are not draining the vegetables after cooking them, we don't want to add too much water; it will make the soup too thin.) Add three tablespoons of olive oil. Bring to a boil and cook over medium heat until all the ingredients are soft.

Remove the pot of boiled vegetables from heat, and without draining the water, use a hand mixer to blend all the ingredients into a vegetable puree. Add the cream cheese to the mixture, and resume cooking over low heat until the cheese melts and mixes well with the vegetables. In order to obtain a more uniform consistency, the mixture may need to be blended again after adding the cheese. Add salt and pepper to taste.

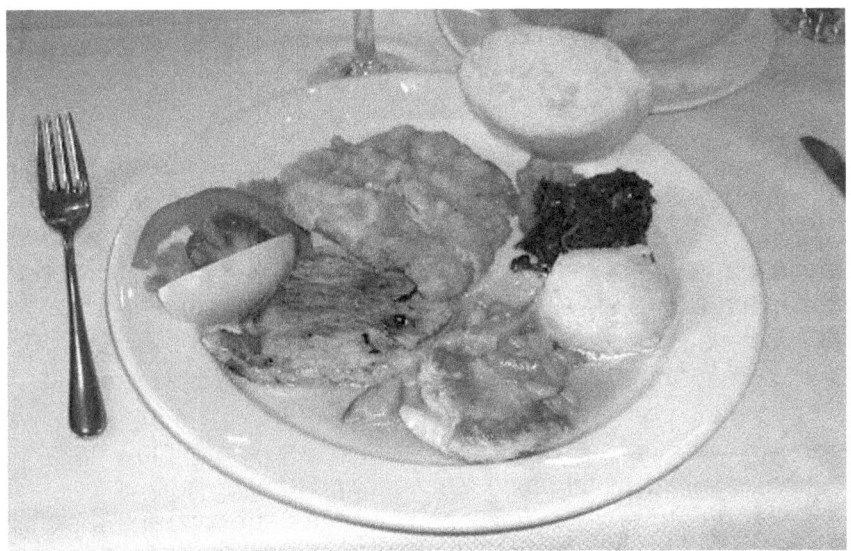

BREADED PORK CUTLETS

Ingredients
6 pork cutlets
1 cup breadcrumbs
garlic powder
2 eggs
olive oil
salt and pepper

Preparation
Sprinkle the pork cutlets with salt, pepper, and garlic powder.

In a mixing bowl, beat the eggs. Dip the cutlets, first into the beaten egg, and then into the breadcrumbs, until they are covered evenly.

Heat olive oil in a skillet over low heat. Add the pork cutlets allowing them to cook on both sides until brown.

Wednesday's Explanations

For today's breakfast, one slice of whole wheat toast provides fiber, and a glass of milk provides calcium. As noted, hard-boiled eggs can be cooked and peeled the night before so that they are ready for breakfast on the go. Eggs are a good source of protein, vitamins, and minerals.

The fruity afternoon snack is quick and light in preparation for a heavier dinner.

The vegetable and cheese soup provides a subtle, simple method for introducing children to vegetables without drawing attention to the fact. Most small children are sensitive to textures and avoid any foods that feel different in the mouth, so increasing the palatability of the vegetables by mixing them with other foods is an ideal way to get children accustomed to greens.

I named the soup after "The Incredible Hulk" at a time when I was trying to convince my toddler to try it. Back then, my youngest son was a big fan of The Hulk, so I invented a story in which the superhero likes this soup so much that he eats enough of it to turn his skin green, and he develops enormous strength and power. I can still see my son's eyes open wide with disbelief as I spooned in the soup without complaints. To this day, "Hulk" soup remains one of his favorites.

Omitting the cheese and making it with only vegetables is a variation on this soup. Carrots can be added to produce an orange, rather than green, final product.

The pork cutlets are a good complement to the soup because they add protein, needed by young and old alike. While adolescents and adults may enjoy and need the pork cutlets to feel satisfied, toddlers and small children may become full with just a bowl of soup for dinner. For a young child, a piece of fruit may accompany the soup to create a complete dinner. Since the soup already contains vegetables, and in order to avoid overeating, we don't need to prepare any side dishes with the pork.

Thursday

Breakfast

HAM AND CHEESE TOAST WITH AN ORANGE

Ingredients
1 slice whole wheat toast
1 slice deli ham
1 slice cheese
1 orange or nectarine
1 glass milk

Preparation
Melt cheese over ham on whole wheat toast, and accompany with an orange or nectarine and a glass of milk.

Afternoon Snack

RASPBERRIES AND COTTAGE CHEESE

Ingredients
2 handfuls fresh raspberries
4 oz. cottage cheese
1 tablespoon sugar
whole wheat crackers

Preparation
Cut the raspberries in half, and mix with one tablespoon of sugar. Add the cottage cheese, and spread over whole wheat crackers.

Dinner: Peppered Salmon and Spinach with Garlic

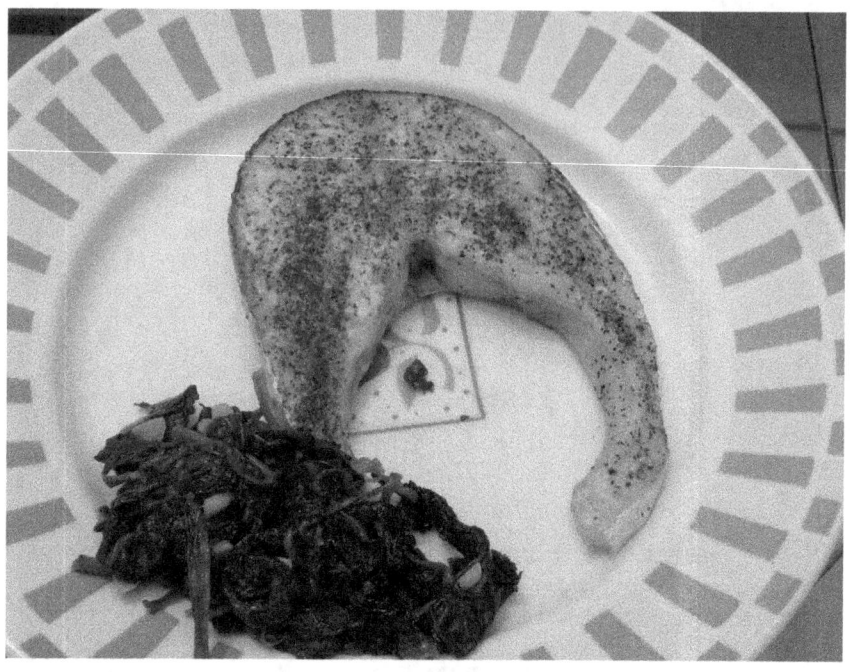

PEPPERED SALMON

Ingredients
1 lb. salmon fillet
olive oil
fresh-ground black pepper

Preparation
Defrost the salmon in the refrigerator. Spread olive oil over both sides, and place the fillet in an oven-safe dish. Pour more olive oil over the top in order to permeate the whole fillet, and allow it to marinate in the refrigerator for a few hours.

*Note: This step can be completed in the morning in order to be ready for cooking at dinnertime.

Add salt to both sides of the salmon fillet, and cover the top with fresh-ground black pepper. Bake in the oven for 15 minutes at 350 degrees.

SPINACH WITH GARLIC

Ingredients
¾ bag spinach
3 garlic cloves
4 tablespoons olive oil

Preparation
Heat four tablespoons of olive oil in a saucepan over medium heat. Mince the garlic and add it to the hot olive oil. After one minute, add the fresh spinach, turning and stirring the leaves until they are soft and covered by oil. It takes about three minutes to cook.

* Note: this is the remainder of the spinach from Monday's dinner.

Thursday's Explanations

Breakfast again provides some protein for long-lasting energy in the morning. Depending on the time of year, the fruit can be an orange or a nectarine. A glass of milk will provide calcium and minerals.

The afternoon snack introduces a fruit with a mild taste and low sugar content. Adding a small amount of sugar and mixing the raspberries with cottage cheese will make the fruit more palatable to children, and will encourage them to continue trying new fruits.

At dinner, salmon provides omega-3 fatty acids and additional calcium to the diet. In addition to being nutritious, fish is always easy to prepare—especially salmon. When the fish starts turning white on the edges and the oil browns slightly, the salmon is ready. Overcooking it may dry the fish and detract from the flavor. It is better to under-cook salmon than to overcook it. Be generous with the fresh-ground black pepper used to cover the fish before putting it in the oven.

Remember to use the three-quarters bag of spinach from Monday's dinner. The special aroma created by the cooking spinach and garlic, combined with the salmon, produces the ambience of a restaurant kitchen that truly whets the appetite.

People who grow up familiar at home with the aromas produced by foods are more likely to consume better-quality meals throughout their entire lives, because children become accustomed to what they are exposed to from an early age. For example, small children from Mexican families are able to eat very spicy foods because they have been introduced to this kind of spice at a young age; they have grown up smelling the hot chili sauce and its ingredients that are used by their parents at home.

By this same token, introducing children to fish after the first year of life will help them learn to enjoy one of the best sources of low-fat protein available. As adults, they will continue to enjoy different varieties of seafood, and they will be less apprehensive to trying new, healthy ingredients.

Friday

Breakfast

ITALIAN SAUSAGE "TACO"

Ingredients
2 Italian sausages
olive oil
½ onion
1 slice whole wheat toast or a whole wheat tortilla
1 glass milk

Preparation
Cut the Italian sausages into small pieces and brown in a skillet, adding a very small amount of olive oil if needed. Mince the onion and cook it with the sausage. Toast a slice of bread or a whole wheat tortilla and pour the sausage and onion mixture in the middle, then fold over.

Pour a glass of milk to drink.

Afternoon Snack

MIXED BERRY YOGURT PUREE

Ingredients
½ bag frozen berries (about 8 oz.)
1 cup plain yogurt

Preparation

Place the frozen berries in a blender and blend until soft. Stir the berry mixture into the yogurt without adding sugar.

Dinner: Chicken Drumsticks and Yellow Rice

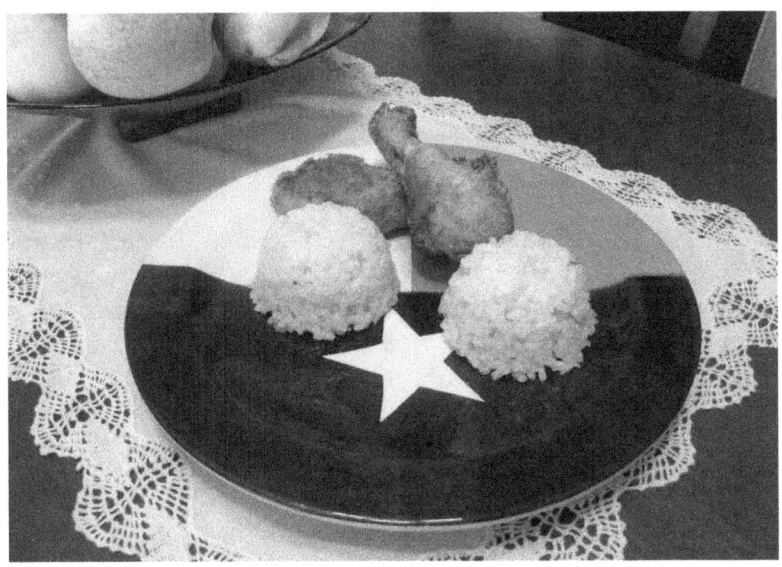

CHICKEN DRUMSTICKS

Ingredients
6–8 chicken drumsticks
olive oil
1 cup breadcrumbs
salt

Preparation
Marinate the chicken drumsticks in olive oil for 20 minutes; add a pinch of salt. Dip the drumsticks in breadcrumbs, and bake them in the oven at 350 degrees for about 50 minutes, turning them as needed.

YELLOW RICE

Ingredients
½ cup rice
½ onion
2 garlic cloves
½ teaspoon saffron
3 tablespoons olive oil
salt

Preparation

Mince the onion and garlic. In a saucepan, heat three table-spoons of olive oil over medium heat, and add the minced onion and garlic. Stir the mixture for about one minute, then add the rice, stirring continuously. Add one and one-half cups of hot water along with the saffron, and continue to stir. Add salt to taste, and cook uncovered over low heat for about 20 minutes. Remove from heat, cover, and let sit for 15 minutes before serving.

Friday's Explanations

Breakfast and snack need no further explanation.

This dinner is fast! The chicken drumsticks cook in the oven without much preparation, and while they are baking, we can prepare the rice, which takes only about 20 minutes to cook.

Yellow rice can be "white" rice if the saffron is not added. Saffron adds flavor, as well as color. It is one of the most aromatic herbs used in Mediterranean-style cooking, and once tasted, it will become a must. We use all of our senses when we eat. Kids appreciate the color of the food they have in front of them as much as the texture and the taste. For some reason, my "picky eater" child always pre-ferred yellow rice and refused to try white rice alleging that he didn't like it. Although I always advise parents not to fall for the "I don't like it" excuse before the food has even been tasted, I have to agree with my son on this one—I also prefer rice with saffron versus white rice.

Saturday

Breakfast/Brunch:

FRIED FRUIT WITH FRENCH TOAST

Ingredients
2 nectarines
1 banana
1 handful blueberries
6 tablespoons olive oil
4 slices whole wheat bread
2 eggs
salt
¼ cup milk
1 glass milk

Preparation
After removing the seed, but leaving on the skin, chop the nectarines. Slice the banana into thin slices. Place both in a saucepan, and add three tablespoons of olive oil. Cover and cook slowly over low heat for five minutes. Add the blueberries. The olive oil will enhance the flavors of the fruits, bringing out all the natural sugars of the banana and the nectarines, while the blueberries complement the mixture by adding a dark color and creamy consistency. When the fruits are soft and blended into a smooth syrup, cooking is complete.

In a mixing bowl, beat the eggs and add a pinch of salt. Mix in the milk. Heat three tablespoons of olive oil in a frying pan over low heat. Dip the slices of whole wheat bread in the egg and milk mixture and place them in the olive oil; flip them once, cooking until brown on both sides.

Serve the French toast with the fruit mixture on top, and pour a glass of milk to drink.

Lunch / Dinner

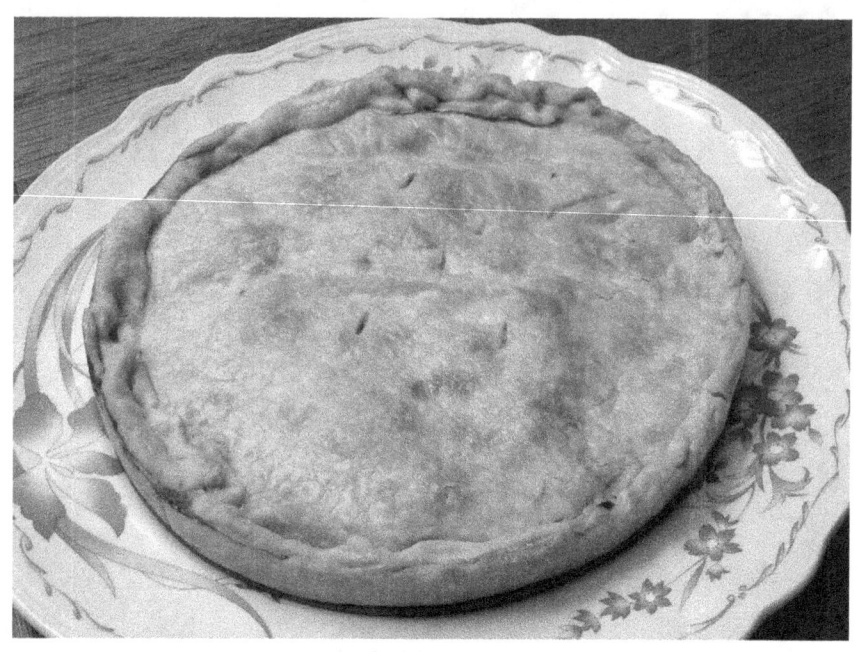

TUNA PIE

Ingredients
2 read½ red bell pepper
½ green bell pepper
1 onion
2 hard-boiled eggs
4 tablespoons olive oil
salt
sugar
1 can white albacore tuna (7 oz.)

Preparation
In a saucepan, heat four tablespoons of olive oil over medium heat. Chop the tomatoes, red pepper, green pepper, and onion, and cook for about 30 minutes. * Add salt and a pinch of sugar if desired. Once the vegetables are cooked to a soft texture, add the hard-

boiled eggs cut into pieces along with the tuna. Allow the mixture to cook for another ten minutes on low heat.

*The half red pepper and half green pepper are remaining from the peppers used in Sunday's recipe for Beef with Vegetables.

Grease the bottom of a round, 9-inch, oven-safe pie pan, and place the lower-layer piecrust in the pie pan. Pour in the tuna-vegetable mixture, and cover with the top-layer piecrust. Fold in the edges sealing the ingredients inside. With a fork, make a few holes in the top crust. Place the dish in the oven, and bake at 350 degrees for about 30 minutes. When the crust is brown all over, the dish is ready.

* Note: To create a sheen, a beaten egg may be brushed over the top crust before placing in the oven.

Saturday's Explanations

Saturday is a special day for most families. Kids are home from school, we generally wake later, and we don't have a structured schedule for the day. Families with children often attend sporting events or run errands and spend much of the day in and out of the house.

I planned a hearty breakfast, including fruits, eggs, bread, and olive oil, that is delicious and easy to prepare. For many, this breakfast is going to be prepared late in the day, and may be considered "brunch" after waking so late.

For the main dish of the day, I chose Tuna Pie, which is as delicious cold as it is right out of the oven. Once it's baked, it can be taken on the road or to events. In its preparation, we are using some of the ingredients leftover from previous days.

Second Sunday

Breakfast

MIXED BERRY YOGURT PUREE

Ingredients
½ bag frozen berries (8 oz.)
1 cup plain yogurt

Preparation
Place the frozen berries in a blender and blend until soft. Stir the berry mixture into the yogurt without adding sugar.

Lunch

HOUSE SALAD

Ingredients
½ head lettuce
1 tomato
1 apple
1 handful fresh blueberries
1 hard-boiled egg
1 can pink salmon (5 oz.)
1 avocado
¼ onion
1 handful fresh raspberries
1 stalk celery
olive oil
vinegar
salt

Preparation
Chop produce, egg, and salmon; mix them in a bowl. Add salt, olive oil, and vinegar to taste.

Sunday's Explanations

Today we are basically "cleaning out the refrigerator" in preparation for another week's groceries and meal planning.

Breakfast includes natural yogurt with frozen berries. The other meal of the day includes a salad composed of some of the leftover ingredients from previous days and a few new ones. This recipe can be fun for the imagination as it involves play with different textures. Mixing fruits with raw vegetables is appetizing, even when the dressing is a simple oil and vinegar. Skip ingredients that are not favorites and add others as preferred.

This salad is a good resource for the busy family. It can be prepared with a moment's notice if necessary. On a particularly busy day, when there is no time to enjoy preparing a full meal, this salad will suffice. It combines all the ingredients the body needs without adding empty calories. There is protein in the salmon and eggs, all the fiber for the day in the fruits and vegetables, and small amounts of carbohydrates as well as many vitamins and minerals.

Chapter 15

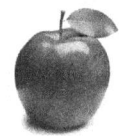 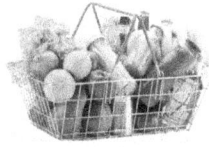 

The Economics of Health

The grocery list provided below includes all the ingredients needed to prepare breakfast, dinner, and an after-school snack for the "One-Week Sample Menu for a Family of Four" (two adults and two children) in the previous chapter. The menu includes a Sunday-to-Sunday "week," plus an extra dish of lentil soup to keep in the freezer for that unpredictable busy day when we may not have time to cook.

Each family, and each member of each family, is going to eat a different amount of food; I designed the menu taking into account a family of four: two adults and two teens. However, if one were to prepare the same amount for a family of two adults and two pre-schoolers, the same quantity of food should last about ten days rather than eight because there will be at least two occasions when the family will have enough leftovers to skip one cooking day.

Based on prices obtained from my local, Austin, Texas, grocery store in March 2012, the cost of the groceries needed to prepare this one-week menu (excluding lunch) totaled $125, taking into account spices and such items that will remain on hand beyond the week. Sticking to this menu plan, a family of two adults and two teens will spend about $480 in one month; a family of two adults and two preschoolers will spend roughly $350.

Does this seem expensive? It will be if, in addition to this grocery list, considerable amounts of money continue to be spent on junk food. However, if the healthy habit of cooking foods from scratch at home replaces the old habit of buying prepared, processed foods and fast food, it will not be expensive. Let's look at it from a different angle. A family of four spending $480 per month for breakfast, dinner, and an after-school snack would be spending a total of $16 per day—only $4 per day, per person. That is actually very reasonable when we compare it to the price of eating out or buying prepared food. Of course, one caveat is that we are not adding to the equation the "cost" of the time needed for grocery shopping and food preparation. Of course, "Time is money," but the payoff is improved health for everyone involved and the opportunity to engage in a family activity that creates traditions.

Shopping List

1 lb. of dried lentils

1 lb. bag of multi-color bowtie pasta

1 lb. of rice

2 leeks

4 carrots

2 blubs of garlic

5 onions

4 potatoes

1 green pepper

1 red pepper

1 bunch of celery

1 head of lettuce

7 tomatoes

1 cucumber

3 zucchini

1 16oz bag of spinach

1 avocado

12 oz of fresh blueberries

12 oz of fresh raspberries

6 apples

6 bananas

6 nectarines

4 oranges (optional if nectarines are not in season)

1 bag of frozen peas and carrots

1 bag of frozen berries

1 bottle of olive oil

1 bottle of vinegar

1 bottle of white wine

salt

pepper

dill weed

garlic powder

1 small bag of sugar

spanish pimenton

saffron

1 container of peanut butter

½ lb. of deli ham, low salt, low nitrates

2 spanish chorizo (optional, instead of Italian sausage for lentils)

4 Italian sausage

2 lb. of rump roast beef

6 pork cutlets

1 lb. of salmon - place in freezer

6-8 chicken drumlets

½ lb. of sliced cheese

1 8 oz. container of cream cheese

1 8 oz. container of cottage cheese

4 yogurt

1 container of plain yogurt

12 eggs

1 pkg. of grated parmesan cheese

2% milk

2 ready-to-bake 9" piecrusts

1 loaf of whole wheat bread

1 box of whole wheat crackers

1 container of bread crumbs

1 can of white Albacore tuna

1 can of pink salmon

© The Step Up Diet
www.DrKatalenas.com

Chapter 16

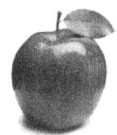 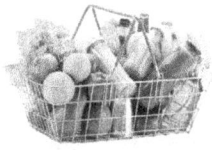 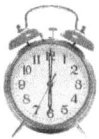

Alternate One-Week
Sample Menu

In order to add variety to the diet I present in this book, I am including here a second one-week sample that can be used either in conjunction with the first week, by itself, or in any order you prefer. There is no particular reason for the order of the days or the recipes; they all present balanced meals from scratch that are easy and fast to prepare.

We are going to begin this alternate menu, like the previous one, by gathering our grocery list and shopping for food on Sunday afternoon, when we have more time to locate all our ingredients.

We start with Sunday evening dinner. The menu is intended for four people, and we are going to consider we have two adults and two teenage children. The amount of food described would need to be adapted for a family with small children; or such a family may end up with enough food prepared to actually last two extra days.

The menu is intended for healthy people who are willing to add structure and variety to their diet. Those with high cholesterol should choose the "low fat" variety of the milk products and consult their doctor before following this or any menu. If you have diabetes, celiac disease, or any chronic disease requiring medical attention, always consult a healthcare professional before making any major changes in your eating habits.

The food we prepare on Sunday is going to last two days: Sunday dinner and Monday dinner.

Sunday

Dinner

MEAT STEW AND POTATOES, LETTUCE AND TOMATO SALAD

Ingredients

2 lbs. beef for stew (cut into small pieces)
2 large onions
4 garlic cloves
½ cup white cooking wine
4 medium potatoes
1 heart of romaine lettuce
2 medium tomatoes
garlic salt
parsley flakes
salt and pepper
2 teaspoons paprika
4 tablespoons olive oil

Preparation

Pour about four tablespoons of olive oil into a pan; it should be enough to cover the bottom of the pan. Heat the oil to a medium heat and add the meat, stirring it to allow cooking all around. We just want the meat to change color from red to grey. The purpose of this first step is to seal the meat with the olive oil, preserving the flavor of the meat throughout the rest of the cooking process. When the meat is ready, take it out of the pan and reserve the oil and the juices from the meat.

Cut the garlic into thin slices and the onions into julianne, thin strips. Add the garlic to the oil first and cook on medium heat for about three minutes. Now add the onions and the meat. Next add salt, pepper, and two teaspoons of paprika and the cooking wine. No added water is needed, as the onions will let out enough juice as they cook.

Allow to cook for one hour on low heat, stirring occasionally, partially covered. Depending on the kind and quality of meat you choose, the cooking process may take longer. Try the meat after one hour to decide if it is ready. When it is ready, the onions will have turned brown in color and the sauce will thicken. After one hour, cover and allow to cool for 15 minutes before serving.

Potatoes

Cut the potatoes in cubes. Sprinkle with olive oil and mix well. Add garlic salt and parsley flakes and mix again.

Place in an oven-safe dish and cook at 350 degrees for 45 minutes, stirring occasionally.

Salad

Cut up one heart of romaine lettuce. Cut two tomatoes into cubes and add to the lettuce. Add a handful of julienned onions (since the amount is small, you can use some of the ones reserved for the meat). Mix all ingredients in a salad bowl; add salt and sprinkle with olive oil and vinegar to taste.

When ready to serve, place two tablespoons of the meat, one tablespoon of the potatoes, and as much salad as desired on a dinner plate. This amount should be enough for an adult. Adjust the amount for small children. If the meat is cooked until tender, it can be cut in very small pieces that can be handled by toddlers.

* Note: Save the leftover meat and potatoes in the refrigerator to use for Monday's dinner.

Monday

Breakfast

1 hard-boiled egg
½ cup grapes
1 glass milk

It is important to remember here the purpose of breakfast. We always want to include some protein; in this case the egg is the main source of protein. We also want to include some fruit, in order to get used to eating fruit with every meal and also to add fiber to the diet, along with vitamins and minerals.

Milk provides additional protein and some needed calcium for growing bones. Adults may prefer a cup of coffee. As far as the fat content of milk, it really depends of your family's needs. A normal growing toddler can take whole milk, while an adult who is trying to lose weight should drink only fat-free milk. But once you have become aware of the different needs of your family, you should be able to make this decision comfortably. Some families just buy 2% milk for everybody, to avoid having to purchase different kinds of the same product.

Afternoon Snack

1 apple (washed, cut, and placed in a bowl)
1 glass milk

Here I want to emphasize the importance of the after-school snack for kids, while stressing that adults may want to skip this meal completely. My advice for adults is to eat just a piece of fruit between lunchtime and dinnertime; a snack as simple and convenient as a piece of fruit can be eaten even during a work break. For kids, an afternoon snack is a time to relax after school and a perfect opportunity for a parent to present them with a variety of fruits they are unlikely to turn down, because they will be hungry. But remember not to ask for their preferences. This only opens a door for a disappointed eater to complain. Children are apt to challenge parents any chance they get, but parents should "choose their battles" wisely.

Because it is usually a simple meal that requires minimal preparation, it can be ready when the child arrives home from school and presented to him or her as a *fait accompli*. Although the child holds the key to whether or not he or she is going to eat what we give them and can certainly refuse to eat, the parent can also refuse to offer options. Don't spend too much time agonizing about it; remember the purpose of this whole exercise is to create habits without engaging in a power struggle. Try your best to offer *your* choice for the day with a smile and lots of love, knowing you are doing the right thing.

Dinner: Meat Stew and Potatoes (left-over from Sunday), with Avocado

Heat the leftovers from Sunday's dinner. Cut ½ avocado in small pieces and serve with the meal.

Tuesday

Breakfast

deli turkey and provolone cheese roll-up
1 glass milk

Remember to buy low-salt, low-nitrate deli meats. You can use chicken or ham if preferred.

Afternoon Snack

2 slices cantaloupe or other melon
1 glass milk

Dinner

GARBANZO BEANS WITH CHICKEN AND TOMATOES

Ingredients
1 can of cooked garbanzo beans (32 oz.)
2 medium tomatoes
1 chicken breast
2 teaspoons paprika
5 tablespoons olive oil
garlic powder
salt and pepper

Preparation
Wash the garbanzo beans with abundant running water and drain well.

In a saucepan place five tablespoons of olive oil. Cut the chicken breast into cubes and sprinkle with salt, pepper, and garlic powder.

Cut the tomatoes into small pieces and add with the paprika. Cook for five minutes and add the garbanzos. Cover and cook for 20 minutes.

Wednesday

Breakfast

whole wheat bread toast with cream cheese
banana
milk

Afternoon Snack

1 apple
milk

Dinner

WHITEFISH AND RICE

Ingredients
4 fillets white fish (tilapia, panga, etc.)
4 garlic cloves
fresh parsley
1 cup rice
½ onion
6 tablespoons olive oil
salt and pepper

Preparation
Chop two garlic cloves and two branches of fresh parsley very fine. Mix with three tablespoons of olive oil. Spread the mixture over the whitefish (both sides) and sprinkle with salt and pepper. Place in an oven-safe dish and cook at 350 degrees for 20 minutes, covered.

Heat one and one-half cups of water. Heat three tablespoons of olive oil in a saucepan. Cut two garlic cloves and ½ onion into small pieces and add it to the oil when it is hot. Stir for about three minutes. Add the rice and stir. Add the water when it is about to boil. Stir for two minutes while cooking on high heat. Turn the heat to low and continue cooking for 20 minutes, half covered. Serve with the fish and sprinkle fresh parsley on top.

Thursday

Breakfast

SCRAMBLED EGGS WITH SPINACH AND MILK

Ingredients
4 eggs
4 handfuls fresh spinach
3 tablespoons olive oil
salt and pepper

Preparation
Beat the eggs, add salt and pepper, and reserve.

In a saucepan add 3 tablespoons of olive oil and heat it. Add the spinach and cook for three minutes, until the leaves are wilted. Add the eggs and stir until cooked.

Afternoon Snack

1 cup seedless grapes
milk

Dinner

VEGETABLE MENESTRA

Ingredients
1 bag frozen peas
1 bag frozen green beans
2 potatoes (cut into small squares)
1 large onion
1 green pepper
1 large carrot (cut into small pieces)
3 garlic cloves
¾ lb. deli ham (thick, cut into squares)
salt and pepper
5 tablespoons olive oil
2 teaspoons paprika

Preparation
Cook the frozen peas and frozen green beans according to directions on the bag, uncovered, until soft. Reserve in the same water.

In a saucepan heat 5 tablespoons of olive oil. Add the garlic cloves, diced. Add the onion (also cut in small pieces), carrot, and green pepper. Cook, stirring frequently, for five minutes. Add the ham and paprika and continue cooking for five more minutes. Now drain the peas and green beans, reserving the cooking water. Add the potatoes and enough cooking water to cover the mixture. Add salt and pepper. Cook on medium heat, covered, for 30 minutes.

Serve in a bowl. This dish should be enough for two days. Leftovers can be reserved for Friday's dinner.

Friday

Breakfast

1 yogurt
1 apple
milk

Afternoon Snack

1 banana
milk

Dinner: Menestra (leftover) with Hard-Boiled Eggs

Heat the leftovers from Thursday's dinner. Cut up two hard-boiled eggs on top.

Saturday

Breakfast

BREAD WITH TOMATO AND MILK

Ingredients
3 rolls French bread
3 tomatoes
3 slices provolone cheese

Preparation
Cut rolls of French bread in half and toast them lightly. Cut the tomatoes in half and spread the inside of the tomato into the bread, squeezing it and discarding the skin. Cut up the slices of provolone cheese into small pieces and place them on top of the tomato. Bake in the oven at 350 degrees for 10 minutes.

Dinner

RUSSIAN SALAD

Ingredients
4 medium potatoes
3 hard-boiled eggs
2 medium carrots
½ bag frozen green peas
1 can tuna (5 oz.)
½ cup olives (cut in small pieces)
olive oil
vinegar
4 tablespoons mayonnaise

Preparation
Cook the carrots (cut into small "wheels") and the frozen peas in boiling water for 15 minutes. Drain and reserve.

Boil the potatoes in water for 20 minutes or until soft. Drain off the water and allow potatoes to cool, then cut into small cubes. Cut up the hard-boiled eggs and add them to the potatoes. Add the carrots, green peas, olives, and tuna (drained). Mix well and sprinkle with olive oil and vinegar. Add four tablespoons of mayonnaise and toss again.

This dish is ideal for Saturday on the go. It can be placed in a small cooler and transported to a picnic area, sports practice, or pool party. It can be served over French bread, inside pita bread, or just on a plate.

Add a few slices of cantaloupe or other melon, and it makes a meal.

Sunday Brunch

SALMON PUDDING
LETTUCE AND SPINACH SALAD
FRUIT SALAD

Ingredients
1 lb. salmon
1 cup white cooking wine
1 cup whipping cream
3 eggs
salt and pepper
2 hearts romaine lettuce
5 oz. fresh spinach
olive oil and vinegar

Preparation
Cut the salmon into small pieces and marinate in the cooking wine for 30 minutes. Place in an oven-safe loaf pan. Beat the eggs, mix in the whipping cream, salt, and pepper, and add the mixture to the salmon. Cook at 350 degrees for 45 minutes. When it solidifies, remove from oven and allow to cool. Remove from oven pan, slice, and serve.

Mix the lettuce and spinach. Add salt and sprinkle with olive oil and vinegar. To make the fruit salad, simply cut up any leftover fruits from the weekly menu and mix them in a bowl.

Chapter 17

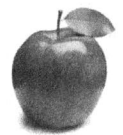 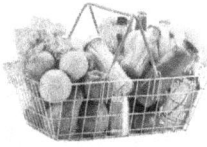 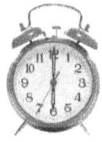

Recipes

These recipes consist of main courses and snacks. The main courses are divided into groups including vegetable dishes, meat dishes, fish dishes, soups and stews, and pastas. Depending on the dish and the time of day, these may be served for breakfast, lunch, or dinner. I recommend serving only one item per meal; this technique decreases the amount of calories by cutting down on "side dishes" while providing a sufficient variety of nutrients all in one dish. It also saves preparation time.

When planning family meals, we must take into account the fact that children don't eat as much as adults; offering only one option per meal and eliminating side dishes will obligate kids to eat what is set before them. The keys to good childhood nutrition are to offer balanced meals, planned in advance, and to refrain from giving too many options at the table.

Main Courses

Vegetable Dishes

FAMILY SALAD

This salad may be served as accompaniment to another dish or on its own; the amount and quality of ingredients qualify it as a meal. Ingredients may be added or subtracted as needed.

Ingredients
1 heart of romaine lettuce
2 small tomatoes, 2 hard-boiled eggs
1 apple
1 (8 oz.) can of whole kernel corn
1 (7 oz.) can of solid white tuna in water
10 black or green olives
3 tablespoons of julienned carrots
virgin olive oil
wine vinegar
salt

Preparation
Cut the heart of romaine lettuce into small strips. Add the tomatoes (peeled and cubed). Add the apple (cut into small pieces). Add the eggs, tuna, corn, olives (chopped), and carrots. Add a pinch of salt, virgin olive oil, and vinegar to taste.

CUCUMBER WITH LEMON SAUCE

Ingredients
2 cucumbers
juice of 1 lemon
2 tablespoons olive oil
fresh parsley
fresh dill
1 teaspoon cornstarch
salt

Preparation
Slice the cucumbers and steam for eight minutes. Mix the lemon juice with two branches of fresh parsley and fresh dill (minced). Add the olive oil and bring to a boil. Mix the cornstarch with a small amount of water to dissolve, and add to the boiling mixture of lemon juice and fresh herbs. Add pinch of salt. Pour mixture over the cooked cucumbers.

CHICKPEA SALAD

Ingredients
1 cup of cooked chickpeas (garbanzos)
2 hard-boiled eggs
2 tomatoes
1 carrot
1 heart of romaine lettuce
1 cup of mayonnaise
½ red bell pepper

Preparation

Shred the romaine lettuce into small pieces and spread on the base of a serving plate. Mix the chickpeas, hard-boiled eggs (sliced), tomatoes (chopped), and carrot (sliced), and spread the mixture over the lettuce. Mix the mayonnaise with the red bell pepper in a blender for a few seconds. Pour over the salad.

SPINACH AND CHEESE OMELET

Ingredients

4 eggs
8 oz. of ricotta cheese
1 tablespoon grated Parmesan cheese
8 oz. fresh spinach
3 tablespoons olive oil
salt and pepper

Preparation

Wash the spinach leaves, dry them, and cut into small pieces. Mix the ricotta cheese and the Parmesan cheese with the spinach. Beat the eggs and add salt and pepper. In an eight-inch frying pan, heat three tablespoons of olive oil. When oil is hot, pour in half of the egg mixture, and allow it to spread and cook over medium heat for about one minute. Flip it over, and allow it to cook for another 20 seconds. Pour half of the spinach and cheese mixture in the middle of the cooked egg, and fold the omelet by bringing the edges to the center. Allow it to cook for about one more minute. Repeat with the remaining egg and spinach-cheese mixture.

Meat Dishes

CHICKEN CROQUETTES

Ingredients

1 chicken breast
6 tablespoons flour
6 tablespoons olive oil
2 1/8 cups milk
1 egg
1 cup breadcrumbs
salt
more olive oil for frying

Preparation

Cut the chicken breast into small cubes, and brown it in two tablespoons of olive oil. Once browned, allow it to cool, and shred. Set shredded chicken aside. In a saucepan, bring approximately four tablespoons of olive oil to medium heat. Slowly add about four tablespoons of the flour while stirring. Add room-temperature milk, and continue to stir while cooking at medium heat for about 15 minutes; the sauce will become thicker as it cooks. After 15 minutes, remove sauce from heat and add browned, shredded chicken breast. Allow it to cool to room temperature. After the mixture is cool, use hands to shape it into balls (croquettes) and set them aside. Beat the egg. Batter the croquettes by dipping them first in the remaining flour, then the egg, and lastly, in the breadcrumbs. Fry in hot olive oil and serve. Add salt to taste.

STEWED CHICKEN

Ingredients

4 chicken legs
1 medium onion
3 medium potatoes
2 garlic cloves
1 bay leaf
1 tablespoon sweet Spanish pimentón
1 small glass cooking wine
olive oil
salt and pepper

Preparation

Marinate chicken legs, with salt and pepper added, for 30 minutes. Brown the legs in hot olive oil for a few minutes. Without removing the chicken from the pan, add the onion (minced), the whole garlic cloves (with the skin), the bay leaf, the Spanish pimentón and the wine, and allow to cook, covered, over medium heat for about 40 minutes. Cut the potatoes in large, thin oval slices, and fry them in olive oil until brown. Serve by spreading the potatoes around the base of the plate and adding the chicken with all its juices on top.

PORK CUTLETS WITH TOMATO SAUCE

Ingredients
2 pork cutlets
1 egg
2 tablespoons flour
1 cup breadcrumbs
2 medium tomatoes
½ onion, ¼ teaspoon sugar
1 teaspoon lemon juice
4 tablespoons olive oil
salt and pepper

Preparation
Pour lemon juice over the pork cutlets, add salt and pepper, and allow them to marinate for 15 minutes. Dip cutlets in flour, then in beaten egg, and lastly in breadcrumbs. Again, dip them in egg and breadcrumbs. Peel and chop tomatoes into cubes and set aside. Chop onion and sauté in one tablespoon of olive oil until transparent. Add cubed tomatoes, salt, pepper, and sugar. Allow tomato sauce to simmer for 15 minutes. Put three tablespoons of olive oil in a frying pan and fry the cutlets until brown. Serve cutlets with tomato sauce poured over the top.

TURKEY WITH CUMIN AND CINNAMON

Ingredients
2 turkey breasts
1 garlic clove
juice of ½ lemon
1 teaspoon cumin
1 teaspoon cinnamon
1 teaspoon paprika
½ cup olive oil
salt and pepper

Preparation
Mix the garlic (minced), lemon juice, cumin, cinnamon, paprika, olive oil, salt, and pepper in a bowl. Blend it using a hand blender. Cut the turkey breasts into cubes, and place them in an oven-safe dish. Pour the blended mixture over the turkey and marinate in the refrigerator for two hours. Cover the dish, and place it in the oven at 250 degrees for 30 minutes. Uncover, and continue cooking for another 30 minutes.

Fish Dishes

Fish preparation is easy and fast and makes for a complete meal. For color and variety, fish may be served with the Family Salad described above, under "Vegetable Dishes."

FRIED WHITEFISH

Any type of white fish, including bass, sea bass, halibut, or flounder, may be prepared according to this recipe.

Ingredients
2–3 whitefish fillets
2 eggs
whole wheat flour
5–6 tablespoons olive oil
juice of 1 lemon
salt

Preparation
Sprinkle the lemon juice over the whitefish fillets, add salt to taste, and marinate for 30 minutes. Heat five to six tablespoons of olive oil in a skillet over medium heat. Beat the eggs. Dip the fish in flour, making sure all sides are covered and shaking off any excess. Next, dip the fish in the beaten eggs, and fry over medium heat until brown on both sides.

GRILLED SWORDFISH

Swordfish, like mahi mahi, has a firm flesh that makes it ideal for the grill.

Ingredients
1 large swordfish fillet
juice of 1 lemon
salt, garlic powder
olive oil

Preparation
Marinate the swordfish fillet in the lemon juice, salt, and garlic powder in the refrigerator for 30 minutes. Heat two tablespoons of olive oil over medium heat on the grill, and add the fish, turning it over after five minutes. (It takes five minutes on each side to obtain a perfectly grilled fish.)

PEPPERED SALMON

Ingredients
1 lb. salmon fillet
olive oil
fresh-ground black pepper

Preparation
Defrost the salmon in the refrigerator. Spread olive oil over both sides, and place the fillet in an oven-safe dish. Pour more olive oil over the top in order to permeate the whole fillet, and allow it to marinate in the refrigerator for a few hours.

* Note: This step can be completed in the morning in order to be prepared for cooking at dinnertime.

Add salt to both sides of the salmon fillet, and cover the top with fresh-ground black pepper. Bake in the oven for 15 minutes at 350 degrees.

WHITEFISH WITH PEPPER SAUCE

Ingredients
2 fillets of white fish
olive oil
parsley
salt
¼ red bell pepper
¼ yellow bell pepper
1/2 cup whipping cream

Preparation
Soak the red and yellow bell peppers (chopped) in a small amount of olive oil until soft. Add the whipping cream, 2 pinches of parsley and salt to taste, and allow it to cook over medium heat for 10 minutes. With a hand blender, blend the mixture of whipping cream and peppers until obtaining a smooth sauce. Heat two tablespoons of olive oil in a saucepan over medium heat, and brown the fish fillets for about 10 minutes. Remove the fish from the heat and serve with the sauce poured over it.

FISH OMELET WITH CHEESE

Ingredients
2 fillets whitefish
olive oil
3 eggs
3 tablespoons white cheese (grated)
salt and pepper
1 tomato

Preparation
Grill the fish fillets in a small amount of olive oil. Beat the eggs, and add salt and pepper. Break the fillets into small pieces, and add them to the beaten egg. Add the cheese. Heat two tablespoons of olive oil in a frying pan until it is very hot, add the mixture of egg, cheese, and fish, and allow it to cook slowly. As the mixture is solidifying, flip the omelet by placing a flat plate on top of the frying pan and turning it over. Cook the omelet on the other side for about five minutes, until the egg starts to brown. It may be served with slices of tomato on top.

WHITEFISH WITH ORANGE SAUCE

Ingredients
2 fillets whitefish
2 oranges
½ cup whipping cream
olive oil
salt and pepper

Preparation
Brown the fish fillets in a small amount of olive oil, and reserve. Squeeze the juice of two oranges, and reserve the pulp of one of them. Heat the orange juice over medium heat, adding the whipping cream gradually, and adding a teaspoon of grated orange pulp. As the sauce cooks slowly, it will thicken slightly. Add salt and pepper to taste. Serve the fish with two teaspoons of orange sauce on top.

TUNA-STUFFED TOMATOES

Ingredients
4 large tomatoes
1 (5 oz.) can of white tuna
1 hard-boiled egg
5 oz. Fontina cheese
8 black olives
olive oil
salt and pepper
¼ cup Parmesan cheese (grated)

Preparation
Cut off the tops of the tomatoes and set aside. Remove the pulp with a spoon, reserve the pulp, and wash the tomatoes with cold water. Face down on a paper towel, allow them to drain. Mix the tuna (drained) with the pulp of the tomatoes, the egg, and the black olives (chopped into small pieces). Add the Fontina cheese (diced), and salt and pepper to the mixture. Stuff the tomatoes with the mixture and replace the tops. Drizzle about three tablespoons of olive oil over them and sprinkle with grated Parmesan cheese. Bake in the oven at 350 degrees for 15 minutes.

Pastas

TOMATO SAUCE

A good pasta dish must begin with a perfect tomato sauce as a base. Considering that many children complain when they see too many vegetables on the plate, a good alternative is to prepare pasta with a tomato sauce that includes some "hidden" vegetables. It may be prepared in advance and kept in the freezer. When pressed for time, simply defrost and serve the kids their favorite pasta as a good dinner solution.

Ingredients
4 large, fresh tomatoes or 1 can tomato puree
½ onion
1 leek
1 small carrot
2 garlic cloves
¼ cup fresh parsley
oregano
basil
olive oil
salt and pepper

Preparation
In a saucepan, heat four tablespoons of olive oil over medium heat. Cut the onion, garlic, leek, fresh parsley, and carrot into small pieces, and heat the vegetables in the oil for about five minutes. Add the tomato puree or the fresh tomatoes (peeled and cut). Cook on low heat for about 30 more minutes. Remove from heat and mix, using a hand blender, until all the ingredients form a sauce of uniform consistency. Add the dried oregano and basil, salt and pepper, and cook over medium heat for an additional 10 minutes. This sauce may be frozen frozen for future use.

PENNE PASTA WITH TOMATOES AND OLIVES

Ingredients

10 ½ oz. penne pasta
1 can tomatoes (peeled)
½ onion
1 garlic clove
10 black olives
10 green olives
3 tablespoons olive oil
oregano
salt and pepper

Preparation

Cook the penne pasta al dente and set aside. In a saucepan, heat three tablespoons of olive oil over medium heat, and sauté the onions (chopped), garlic (minced), and canned tomatoes (chopped). Cook slowly for 15 minutes. Add the olives (cut into small pieces) and oregano, salt and pepper. Cook for 10 more minutes. Add the cooked pasta and serve.

PASTA SALAD

Ingredients
10 ½ oz. multicolor bow tie pasta
3 ½ oz. cooked deli ham (cubed)
1 tomato
4 leaves lettuce
2 cucumbers
10 black olives
1/3 cup mayonnaise
salt
fresh parsley

Preparation
Cook the pasta al dente, with salt to taste, and reserve. Cool pasta by rinsing in cool water. Mix the ham, lettuce, tomato, cucumbers, and olives (all chopped into small pieces). Add the mayonnaise and mix with the cooked pasta. Sprinkle with small bits of minced fresh parsley and serve.

PASTA WITH OYSTER MUSHROOMS

Ingredients
16 oz. multicolor bow tie pasta
1 cup oyster mushrooms
8 oz. whipping cream
¼ cup parsley
2 garlic cloves
3 tablespoons olive oil
salt and pepper

Preparation
Cook pasta in boiling water until tender. Drain and reserve. Sauté mushrooms with garlic (minced) in about three tablespoons of olive oil over medium heat for about five minutes. Add the parsley (minced), whipping cream, two tablespoons of water, salt and pepper, and cook for approximately five minutes. Pour the sauce over the pasta and serve.

Snacks

What Is the Perfect Snack?

One day in the office, a patient asked me this question: "What suggestions do you have for a perfect snack for my kids?" It sounds like a straightforward question that should have a simple answer, but my reply was far longer and more complicated than my patient expected.

Here is my take on snacks: Snacks are small portions of food eaten between meals in order to curb the hunger sensation produced by hours of food deprivation. For a snack to be perfect in my book, it must be:

— nutritious
— light
— easy to prepare
— low in cost

The timing of the snack is also important. We must define what we mean when we say, "It is snack time," because this phrase may have different significance depending on whom we are talking to. Day-care centers often use snack time as a break between activities, and they offer small amounts of food to children every couple of hours. This practice has many detrimental effects on toddlers and older preschool kids. It spoils the main meals of the day since, as a result of snacking, children lack a proper appetite when they come to the table, and it creates a certain amount of distension in the stomach that, with time and training, children learn to expect. A child who eats small meals all day long for years will grow into an adult who needs to eat constantly. As I have mentioned many times, eating small snacks throughout the day also ends up creating the habit of "emotional eating" whereby a person ends up eating when bored or under stress.

In my opinion, kids need *one* after-school snack. Why? Because most schools offer lunch at noon—or earlier—and dinnertime may be more than six hours away. Transitions tend to make us hungry; finishing the school day, riding a bus and arriving home counts as a transition, and it warrants a good snack.

Now I can share my idea of a good snack: a piece of fruit and a glass of milk.

This snack meets all of the aforementioned criteria of an ideal snack, and it is easy to duplicate. If the child is a teenager able to burn large amounts of food, provide *two pieces of fruit* and a glass of milk.

Here are some ideas of how to make more sophisticated combinations with very basic ingredients, and to obtain the same results as far as simplicity and easy preparation are concerned.

For Toddlers (one to two years of age)

At this age, children tend to become picky eaters, and they select their preferences based on how food feels in the mouth. Texture, color, and presentation play an important role. Therefore, disguising those factors makes snack time more successful. It also provides an opportunity to introduce a couple of servings of fruit for the day.

FRUIT PUREE

Ingredients
½ banana
½ apple
1 nectarine
1 graham cracker
the juice of ½ orange

Preparation
Mix all ingredients together, and with a hand blender, blend for a few seconds.

For Older Children (over two years of age)

STRAWBERRY MOUSSE

Ingredients
1 lb. fresh or frozen strawberries
2 cups whipping cream
½ cup sugar
2 egg whites

Preparation
Refrigerate small glass cups in preparation for serving. In a blender, blend the strawberries with half of the sugar. In a separate bowl, beat the egg whites until they are fluffy while adding the remaining sugar. In another bowl, whip the cream until soft, then slowly mix in the blended strawberries and sugar, and mix in the whipped egg whites and sugar. Serve in small glass cups.

PEARS AND CHEESE

Ingredients
2 pears
2 tablespoons blue cheese
2 tablespoons plain cream cheese
lemon juice
2 teaspoons honey
2 tablespoons crushed walnuts

Preparation
Cut pears in half and core them, removing the center with a small scoop. Pour lemon juice over the pears to avoid oxidation and color changes. In a bowl, combine the two cheeses, blending them with a fork. Add the honey and nuts to the mixture. Pour the mixture inside the center hole of the pears.

CRACKERS WITH RASPBERRIES AND CHEESE

Ingredients
whole wheat crackers
white cream cheese
3 ½ oz. raspberries
1 teaspoon sugar

Preparation
Cut raspberries in half and mix in sugar. Spread cream cheese over crackers and pour raspberries on top.

PEACH AND STRAWBERRY SOUP

Ingredients
2 peaches
3 ½ oz. fresh or frozen strawberries
1 cup orange juice
1 tablespoon peach preserves

Preparation
Peel and chop the peaches, removing the pit. Blend the peaches, orange juice, and peach preserves into a soup. Refrigerate for a few minutes, then serve in small glasses.

BANANAS WITH YOGURT

Ingredients
2 bananas
1 tablespoon olive oil
1 tablespoon lemon or lime juice
1 plain yogurt
2 tablespoons honey

Preparation
Cut the bananas into small pieces, and brown them in olive oil for about five minutes. Remove them from heat. Pour in the lemon or lime juice. In a separate bowl, combine the plain yogurt and honey. Pour over the cooked bananas and serve.

SWEET APPLES WITH CINNAMON

Sweet apples can be served warm or cooled in the refrigerator depending on the outside temperature and the time of year. They make a good afternoon snack for little ones, as well as a good companion to pork dishes and fish.

Ingredients
2 green apples
3 tablespoons sugar
1 tablespoon butter
1 cinnamon stick

Preparation
Core and cut the apples into cubes. Place them in a pan and barely cover with water. Add the butter, sugar, and cinnamon stick, and cook slowly for 15 minutes.

Chapter 18

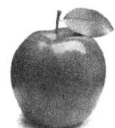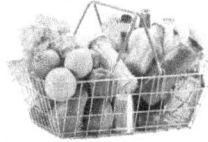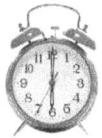

School Lunch from Scratch

When it comes to reversing the obesity epidemic in the United States, schools are in a unique, potentially advantageous position: They have the opportunity not only to teach children how to eat right but to present them with healthy food at a time of day when they are hungry. After four hours of schoolwork, most kids feel hungry and thirsty by the time they walk into the school cafeteria. Additionally, as when kids participate in any group activity, they tend to imitate behaviors and to try to impress each other. If schools were to present them only with healthy food made from scratch on the school premises, kids would have no other option but to eat it. The first day, they might decide they don't like what is offered, and many might leave the cafeteria hungry. But it wouldn't take very long for students to discover that their best bet is to try what they are given and make the best out of the situation. If the same strategy is followed at home, very soon even the pickiest eater will be on his or her way to discovering new and exciting meals that nourish both body and mind.

However, the school lunch program as it stands today presents kids with options. We allow children to choose, based on what they like, at an age when they don't have enough knowledge (or sense) to make informed choices. Like in any other aspect of life, eating behavior must be modeled by adults in order for children to eventually be able to choose. We don't get up in the morning and give children the option whether to go to school or to stay home and play video games. It would be absurd to do so. We don't negotiate this important part of their lives; neither should the learning of good eating habits be negotiated. Just as we do when it comes to academics, parents and schools must join forces to accomplish this goal.

Toward this end, I offer a sample lunch menu intended to feed ten school-aged children. Just to get an idea of costs, I went to my local grocery store and I figured out how much it would take to purchase the ingredients for this menu for one week. I came up with $115.61 per week for ten kids, or $23.12 per day; or $2.31 per plate. These figures don't take into account the overhead cost related to food preparation, but we also have to consider that schools get bulk rates when buying large amounts of groceries.

With a mind toward finances, I included in this menu legumes, an inexpensive plant source of protein that is rich in nutrients. Most legumes originated in the Americas and were introduced into Europe as a result of Christopher Columbus's and others' discov-

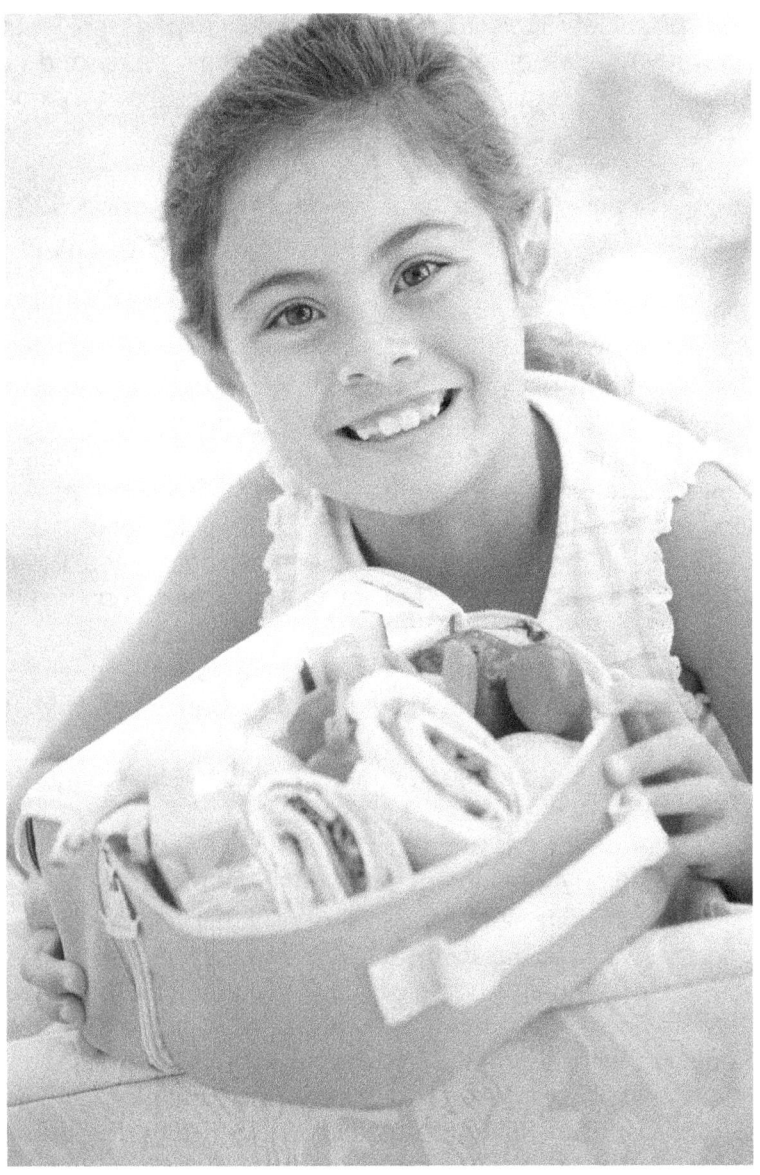

eries. Other legumes have been eaten in Europe and the Middle East for thousands of years. There was a time, during the Middle Ages, when there was not enough meat to go around, that legumes were a staple source of protein. Only the rich could afford meat, and the poor, who had to eat legumes, ended up healthier than the kings and aristocrats who were plagued by gout, obesity, and heart disease. That age-old epidemic is back and is affecting every stratum of society indiscriminately. Nutrition experts are pointing out the advantages of legumes such as beans, peas, and lentils as sources of essential amino acids, minerals, and antioxidants, without saturated fats or cholesterol.

This menu also introduces into school lunches Spanish pimentón (Spanish paprika) as a condiment. It is natural, salt- and preservative-free, and it provides just enough flavor to appeal to kids. It is made with dried red peppers alone. Saffron is another condiment that, being obtained from flowers, provides a natural way of enhancing and blending flavors.

It is important not only that food is of good quality, but that it is served in a calm, soothing environment. Eating time should be quiet and relaxing. Over the years, I've had many opportunities to visit my children's school cafeteria to share lunch with them. The experience was disturbing, not only because of the poor quality of food offered, but because of the level of noise and chaos. From the busy lunch line, we moved to a noisy table where we had just a few minutes to empty our trays and get back to business.

There is an international movement afoot known as "Slow Food." Originally founded in Italy in 1986 by Carlo Petrini, in 1989, Slow Food was developed into a nonprofit association. Over the years, it has gained representation in more than 150 countries and has over 100,000 members. The notion of Slow Food came about as a counterpoint to the fast-food industry. In other words, Slow Food is the antonym to fast food in a gastronomic dictionary.

Slow Food refers not only to the *quality* of the food we eat, but also to the *way* we eat it. If fast food means easy to access to low-priced, poor-quality ingredients that are eaten on the run, Slow Food represents quality food that is prepared at home from scratch and enjoyed with in a leisurely way, mindfully. As when discussing the Mediterranean diet, I don't believe a single ingredient or a single cooking style epitomizes the Slow Food idea. It represents, rather, a holistic attitude toward life that goes beyond eating, just as our fast-food culture is representative not only of food prepared a certain way, but of a society that seeks short-run comfort and convenience despite the long-term negative consequences.

Allow me to illustrate my experience with the Slow Food culture taken as a whole. A few years ago, during one of my summer trips to Spain, my mother informed me they had just opened a new giant grocery store in town. "It is like the ones you have in America," she said, "with everything under one roof." I imagined something like a big Wal-Mart, which my mother enjoys visiting during her frequent trips to the States. Off we went to the store in my father's old car that, having a standard transmission, made for a bumpy ride as we drove through town and I kept forgetting to press the clutch.

When we arrived, I had to park on the lot located across the street because the store's small lot was full. After walking to the entrance of the store, we realized there were no shopping carts in sight. That is because they don't keep the shopping carts by the entrance of the store, but on an island located in the middle of the parking lot. My mother and I retraced our steps through the lot, picked out a cart, and walked back to the store. It didn't take me very long to notice that I had selected a defective cart; this one kept turning stubbornly to the right, and I had to apply considerable force to keep it from going around in circles.

Once inside the store, while my mother was happily showing me the different aisles and the many choices offered, I was sweating from fighting with my obstinate shopping cart. No longer paying attention to the wonders of the establishment, I was noticing how incredibly hot it was. When I made the comment to my mother, who didn't seem to feel at all uncomfortable, she reminded me that in America, our bodies have forgotten how to adjust to changes in the environment because we are used to maintaining a constant temperature. "Besides," she explained, "it is very expensive to keep the AC low in such a large building."

When we finally finished shopping and waiting forever at the cashier, we ventured back outside into the heat of summer. We pushed the cart uphill through the parking lot, up the curve, down the curve, across the street and to the car. After unloading the groceries, I returned the cart to the center of the lot. I imagined the cool air on my shining face, my hair sticking to my makeup, as I would pump up the AC on my drive back to the house. I then remembered I was driving my dad's old car without air conditioning. With my mind fixed on getting home as soon as possible, I rolled down the window allowing the hot air and pollution into the car, and I developed a headache.

When we arrived home from what my mother described as a "fun and productive trip to the grocery store," I was completely exhausted and about to pass out. Meanwhile, my 73-year-old mother helped me carry all our shopping bags into the house and proceeded to put things away while asking me to go and rest because, she said, "Honey, you look pale." A few minutes later, when my aunt came to the door, the two of them decided to go for a walk since it was "such a nice day, and we haven't done anything today."

My story illustrates how differently we perceive daily life based on our customs. For me, a trip to the grocery store involves driving in a nice air-conditioned car and parking as closely as possible to the entrance, even if I have to circle the lot a few times. The carts are right inside the store, or near the entrance, and the ride is smooth. There are plenty of cashiers open to minimize waiting, and some nice youngster pushes my cart back to the car and helps me put the groceries away. I park in my garage, which is next to the kitchen, and all physical effort is kept to a minimum—no sweating involved.

What does this have to do with the Slow Food concept? Everything! Slow Food implies a slower-paced life, taking it easy, not stressing over but instead tolerating inconveniences with a great dose of patience. It goes far beyond the type of food we consume.

Here, in this book, I only introduce the concept. It would take an entire other volume to fully explain how to slow down our way of life. For now, let's concentrate on the eating part. We need to provide kids at school with a calm environment where they can chew their food and enjoy the experience. The deafening cacophony created in a school cafeteria by hundreds of children screaming at each other while eating poor-quality food is not what their brains need in the middle of the school day.

MONDAY

CHICKEN WITH VEGETABLES

Ingredients
10 pieces of chicken
6 medium potatoes
5 carrots
3 tomatoes
3 zucchini
1 large onion
3 garlic cloves
1 green bell pepper
1/2 cup olive oil
salt and pepper
3 teaspoons Spanish pimentón

Preparation
In a large pot, heat half a cup of olive oil over medium heat. Mince the onion and garlic, and add it to the olive oil when it begins to heat. Add the chicken, and allow it to brown slightly on both sides. Add three teaspoons of Spanish pimentón and stir. Chop the potatoes, tomatoes, carrots, and bell pepper, and add them to the chicken, stirring and mixing all ingredients. Add one cup of water, and allow the mixture to cook on low for about half an hour. Chop the zucchini, add it to the pot, and continue to cook on low heat for another half hour. Add salt and pepper to taste.

This dish may be served with a slice of whole wheat bread, one cup of milk, and an apple.

TUESDAY

FISH STEW

Ingredients
6 potatoes
1 large onion
1 red bell pepper
5 celery stalks
3 garlic cloves
2 lbs. whitefish (cod, orange roughy, tilapia)
salt and pepper
3 teaspoons Spanish pimentón
1 envelope or 1 tsp of saffron
1/2 cup olive oil

Preparation
Chop the potatoes, red bell pepper, and celery stalks, and set aside. Heat half a cup of olive oil in a saucepan over medium heat. Mince the onion and garlic, add them to the olive oil, and cook until the onion is transparent. Add the chopped potatoes, red bell pepper, and celery, and stir. Cut the fish into small pieces, and add them to the mixture. Add enough water to slightly cover the ingredients. Add salt, pepper, three teaspoons of Spanish pimentón and one envelope of saffron. Allow it to cook uncovered on low heat for about 45 minutes.

Serve the dish with a slice of whole wheat bread, a glass of milk, and an orange.

WEDNESDAY

GARBANZO BEANS WITH CHICKEN AND BEEF

Ingredients

2 lbs. dried garbanzo beans
5 chicken thighs (cut into small pieces)
1 lb. beef (cubed)
4 carrots
4 potatoes
1 large onion
2 leeks
3 garlic cloves
1/2 cup olive oil
salt and pepper
1 pinch of saffron

Preparation

* Note: Garbanzo beans may be soaked in water overnight to soften; this way, they will cook more quickly.

In a large pot, heat half a cup of olive oil over medium heat. Mince the onions and garlic, and add them to the olive oil. When the onions are transparent, add the potatoes, carrots, and leeks, all cut into small pieces, stirring well. Add the chicken and beef, and stir them into the vegetables. Cover and allow to cook over medium heat for five minutes. Add the garbanzo beans and enough water to cover all the ingredients. Add salt, pepper, and saffron, and allow the mixture to cook over low heat for two to three hours. Serve in a bowl with a slice of whole wheat bread, a glass of milk, and an apple.

*Note: Depending on the type and origin, garbanzo beans can take a long time to cook. They are ready when they are soft.

THURSDAY

BEEF STEW

Ingredients

2 lbs. beef (cubed)
4 potatoes
1 onion (minced)
1 green bell pepper
4 celery stalks
4 tomatoes
3 garlic cloves (minced)
1/3 cup of rice
1/2 cup of olive oil
3 teaspoons Spanish pimentón
salt and pepper

Preparation

In a saucepan, heat the olive oil over medium heat, and add the minced onion and garlic. Chop the potatoes, bell pepper, tomatoes, and celery, and add them to the saucepan. Stirring well, add the meat and three teaspoons of Spanish pimentón. Cover, and allow the mixture to cook over low heat for another 10 minutes. Continuing to stir, add the rice and enough water to cover all the ingredients. Allow it to cook, uncovered, on low heat for 45 to 60 minutes.

Serve with a slice of whole wheat bread, a glass of milk, and half a cup of grapes.

FRIDAY

NAVY BEANS WITH VEGETABLES AND PASTA

Ingredients
2 lbs. navy beans or white beans
2 leeks
4 carrots
large onion
3 garlic cloves
½ cup of pasta (small shells)
3 hard-boiled eggs
1/3 cup olive oil
3 teaspoons Spanish pimentón
salt and pepper

Preparation
Heat one-third cup of olive oil over medium heat. Mince onion and garlic and add to the saucepan. Chop the leeks and carrots, and add them while stirring well. Add three teaspoons of Spanish pimentón and the navy beans. Add enough water to cover the ingredients and cook, partially covered, on low heat for two hours. Add the pasta along with salt and pepper to taste, and allow the mixture to cook for 20 more minutes. Chop the hard-boiled eggs and sprinkle over the soup. Serve this dish with a slice of whole wheat bread, a glass of milk, and one nectarine or orange.

This school lunch model takes into account the limited amount of time allowed for lunch: it includes only one dish per meal—a dish that is easy to cook and serve even for a large number of kids—accompanied by bread, milk, and fruit. As for creating the calm environment in which it would be served, I'll have to leave the logistics to school administrators and other experts.

School administrators, teachers, and parents must agree on the importance of the task and join together to create a new generation of healthy eaters. We can do it, and if we all agree on the basics, it won't be that difficult. We don't need to revisit the obesity epidemic affecting our society, or be reminded that our kids are going to have shorter life spans as a consequence. As parents, we are aware of the problem. We just need a little help solving it. We don't need a degree in economics to understand the financial implications of having our coming generations plagued with chronic diseases from an early age. Granted, resources are limited, but we must take care of our children now if we want them to take care of our future. We can do it.

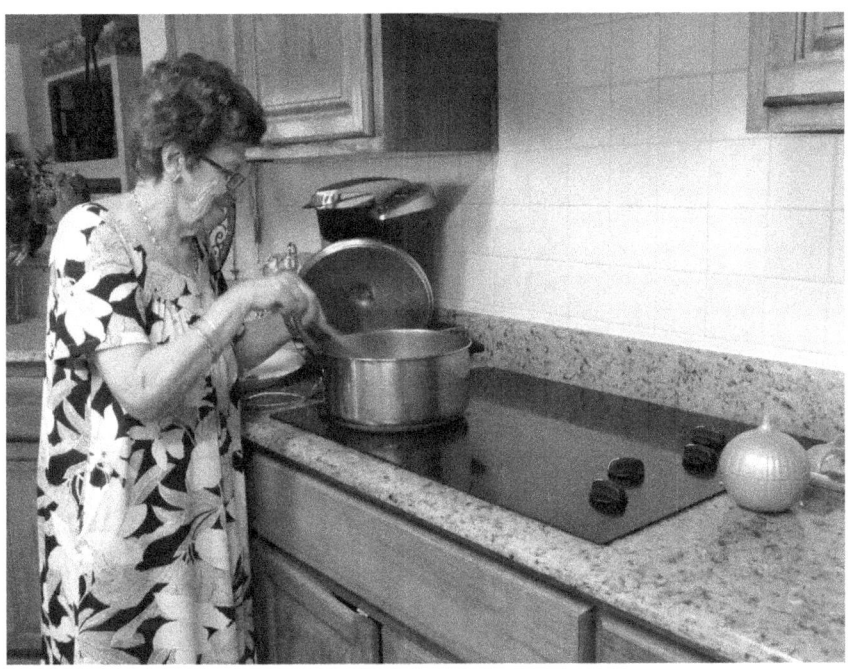

The best cook in the world; my mother Angeles Muñiz

References

Ascherio, Alberto, MD, DrPH; Martijn B. Katan, PhD; Peter L. Zock, PhD; Meir J. Stampfer, MD, DrPH; and Walter C. Willett, MD, DrPH. "Trans Fatty Acids and Coronary Heart Disease." *New England Journal of Medicine* 340 (June 1999): 1994–98.

Ball, Shauna D., MS; Kelly R. Keller, MS; Laurie J. Moyer-Mileur, PhD; Yi-Wen Ding, MS; David Donaldson, MD; and W. Daniel Jackson, MD. "Prolongation of Satiety after Low Versus Moderately High Glycemic Index Meals in Obese Adolescents." *Pediatrics: Official Journal of the American Academy of Pediatrics* 111, no. 3 (March 2003): 488–94.

Byers, Tim, MD, MPH. "Hardened Fats, Hardened Arteries?" *New England Journal of Medicine* 337 (November 1997): 1544–45.

Daniels, Stephen R., MD, PhD; Frank R. Greer, MD, and the Committee on Nutrition. "Lipid Screening and Cardiovascular Health in Childhood." *Pediatrics: Official Journal of the American Academy of Pediatrics* 122, no. 1 (July 2008): 198–208.

Feart, Catherine, PhD; Cecilia Samieri, MPH; Virginie Rondeau, PhD; Helene Amieva, PhD; Florence Portet, MD, PhD; Jean-Francois Dartingues, MD, PhD; Nikolaos Scarmeas, MD; Pascale Barberger-Gateau, MD, PhD. "Adherence to a Mediterranean Diet: Cognitive Decline and Risk of Dementia." *Journal of the American Heart Association* 302, no. 6 (2009): 638–48.

Greer, Frank R., MD; Nancy F. Krebs, MD; and the Committee on Nutrition. "Optimizing Bone Health and Calcium Intakes of Infants, Children and Adolescents." *Pediatrics: Official Journal of the American Academy of Pediatrics* 117, no. 2 (February 2006): 578–85.

Gu, Yian, PhD; Jeri W. Nieves, PhD; Yaakov Stern, PhD; Jose A. Luchsinger, MD, MPH; Nikolaos Scarmeas, MD, MS. "Food

Combination and Alzheimer Disease Risk: A Protective Diet." In "Archives Neurology," *Journal of the American Heart Association* 67, no. 6 (2010): 699–706.

Hassink, Sandra Gibson, MD. *A Clinical Guide to Pediatric Weight Management and Obesity.* Philadelphia: Lippincott Williams & Wilkins, 2007.

Jago, Russell, PhD; Joanne S. Harrell, PhD; Robert G. McMurray, PhD; Sharon Edelstein, ScM; Laure El Ghormli, MSc; and Stanley Bassin, EdD. "Prevalence of Abnormal Lipid and Blood Pressure Values among an Ethnically Diverse Population of Eighth-Grade Adolescents and Screening Implications." *Pediatrics: Official Journal of the American Academy of Pediatrics* 117, no. 6 (June 2006): 2065–73.

Johnson, Rachel K., PhD, MPH, RD, Chair; Lawrence J. Appel, MD, MPH, FAHA; Michael Brands, PhD, FAHA; Barbara V. Howard, PhD, FAHA; Michael Lefevre, PhD, FAHA; Robert H. Lustig, MD; Frank Sacks, MD, FAHA; Lyn M. Steffen, PhD, MPH, RD, FAHA; and Judith Wylie-Rosett, EdD, RD; on behalf of the AHA Nutrition Committee of the Council on Nutrition, Physical Activity, and Metabolism and the Council on Epidemiology and Prevention. "Dietary Sugars Intake and Cardiovascular Health: A Scientific Statement from the American Heart Association." *Circulation: Journal of the American Heart Association* 120, no. 11 (2009): 1011–20.

Katan, Martijn B., PhD; and David S. Ludwig, MD. "Extra Calories Cause Weight Gain—but How Much?" *Journal of the American Medical Association* 303, no. 1 (January 2010): 65–66.

Kleinman, Ronald, MD, ed. *Pediatric Nutrition Handbook*, 6th ed. American Academy of Pediatrics, 2009.

Lichtenstein, Alice H., DSc; Lynne M. Ausman, DSc; Susan M. Jalbert, MLT; and Ernst J. Schaefer, MD. "Effects of Different Forms of Dietary Hydrogenated Fats on Serum Lipoprotein Cholesterol Levels." *New England Journal of Medicine* 340 (June 1999): 1933–40.

Mellanby, Edward, on behalf of the Medical Research Council, Great Britain. "Experimental Rickets." *Special Report Series* 61 (1921): 1–78.

Misra, Madhusmita, MD, MPH; Danièle Pacaud, MD; Anna Petryk, MD; Paulo Ferrez Collett-Solberg, MD; and Michael Kappy, MD, PhD; on behalf of the Drug and Therapeutics Committee of the Lawson Wilkins Pediatric Endocrine Society. "Vitamin D Deficiency in Children and Its Management: Review of Current Knowledge and Recommendations." *Pediatrics: Official Journal of the American Academy of Pediatrics* 122, no. 2 (August 2008): 398–417.

Nelson, Jennifer, MS, RD, CNSD; Karen E. Moxness, MS, RD; Michael D. Jensen, MD; and Clifford E. Gastineau, MD, PhD. *Mayo Clinic Diet Manual: A Handbook of Nutrition Practices*, 7th ed. St. Louis: Mosby Year-Book, 1994.

Pretlow, Robert A., MD, MSEE, FAAP. *Overweight: What Kids Say.* Seattle: CreateSpace, 2010.

Rose, Susan R., MD; Maria G. Vogiatzi, MD; and Kenneth C. Copeland, MD. "A General Pediatric Approach to Evaluating a Short Child." *Pediatrics in Review* 26 (November 2005): 410–20.

Scarmeas, Nikolaos, MD; Jose A. Luchsinger, MD; Nicole Schupf, PhD; Adam M. Brickman, PhD; Stephanie Cosentino, PhD; Ming X. Tang, PhD; Yaakov Stern, PhD. "Physical Activity, Diet and Risk of Alzheimer Disease." *Journal of the American Heart Association* 302, no. 6 (2009): 627–37.

Sperling, Mark A., MD. *Pediatric Endocrinology.* 3rd ed. Philadelphia: Saunders Elsevier, 2008.

Thienprasert, Alice, PhD; Suched Samuhaseneetoo, PhD; Kathryn Popplestone, BSc; Annette L. West, BSc; Elizabeth A. Miles, PhD; and Philip C. Calder, PhD. "Fish Oil N-3 Polyunsaturated Fatty Acids Selectively Affect Plasma Cytokines and Decrease Illness in Thai Schoolchildren: A Randomized, Double Blind, Placebo-Controlled Intervention Trial." *Journal of Pediatrics* 154, no. 3 (March 2009): 391–95.

Wagner, Carol L., MD; and Frank R. Greer, MD; and the Section on Breastfeeding and Committee on Nutrition. "Prevention of Rickets and Vitamin D Deficiency in Infants, Children and Adolescents." *Pediatrics: Official Journal of the American Academy of Pediatrics* 122, no. 5 (November 2008): 1142–52.

Welsh, Jean A., MPH, RN; Andrea Sharma, PhD, MPH; Jerome L. Abramson, PhD; Viola Vaccarino, MD, PhD; Cathleen Gillespie, MS; and Miriam B. Vos, MD, MSPH. "Caloric Sweetener Consumption and Dyslipidemia among U.S. Adults." Journal of the American Heart Association 303, no. 15 (2010): 1490–97.

Index

Recipes

Shopping List

1 lb. of dried lentils
1 lb. bag of multi-color bowtie pasta
1 lb. of rice
2 leeks
4 carrots
2 blubs of garlic
5 onions
4 potatoes
1 green pepper
1 red pepper
1 bunch of celery
1 head of lettuce
7 tomatoes
1 cucumber
3 zucchini
1 16oz bag of spinach
1 avocado
12 oz of fresh blueberries
12 oz of fresh raspberries
6 apples
6 bananas
6 nectarines
4 oranges (optional if nectarines are not in season)
1 bag of frozen peas and carrots
1 bag of frozen berries
1 bottle of olive oil
1 bottle of vinegar
1 bottle of white wine
salt

pepper
dill weed
garlic powder
1 small bag of sugar
spanish pimenton
saffron
1 container of peanut butter
½ lb. of deli ham, low salt, low nitrates
2 spanish chorizo (optional, instead of Italian sausage for lentils)
4 Italian sausage
2 lb. of rump roast beef
6 pork cutlets
1 lb. of salmon - place in freezer
6-8 chicken drumlets
½ lb. of sliced cheese
1 8 oz. container of cream cheese
1 8 oz. container of cottage cheese
4 yogurt
1 container of plain yogurt
12 eggs
1 pkg. of grated parmesan cheese
2% milk
2 ready-to-bake 9" piecrusts
1 loaf of whole wheat bread
1 box of whole wheat crackers
1 container of bread crumbs
1 can of white Albacore tuna
1 can of pink salmon

www.ingramcontent.com/pod-product-compliance
Lightning Source LLC
Chambersburg PA
CBHW070638290526
45790CB00001B/134